'*The Spirit of the Drive* is grippingly written and takes the reader on an intricate journey. Indeed, the subject matter presented so seemingly effortlessly is complex and it contains much material in terms of neurobiology and psychoanalytic theories. This is cleverly done because it requires a great deal of knowledge, thought and experience. The notes are thorough and very comprehensive. I find this book engaging and stimulating. It is thought-provoking and it is both instructive and informative.'

Antoine Mooij, *MD, PhD,*
emeritus professor at Utrecht University,
the Netherlands

'What if a most experienced clinician wrote a book that connects ongoing debates in the neurosciences with key insights from psychoanalysts like Freud and Lacan, and applied it to contemporary clinical problems? Well, that book is *The Spirit of the Drive in Neuropsychoanalysis*, a remarkable achievement by Mark Kinet. Read it!'

Stijn Vanheule, *PhD,*
clinical psychologist and professor of psychoanalysis
and clinical psychology at Ghent University, Belgium

'The author manages to bring together different psychoanalytic schools of thought with neuroscience as a backbone. The book is rooted in a lifetime of psychoanalytic practice and publishing. It is written in a lucid, at times poetic language. Amazingly original and enriching!'

Rudi Vermote, *MD, PhD,*
emeritus professor at KU Leuven, Belgium

The Spirit of the Drive in Neuropsychoanalysis

The Spirit of the Drive in Neuropsychoanalysis gives a concise introduction to the basics of neuropsychoanalysis, both theoretically and clinically.

Kinet uses a colloquial approach to discuss topics such as the dynamic and descriptive unconscious, dream theory, homeostasis, affect and awareness, pleasure and *jouissance*, the signifier and the drive. Throughout the volume, Kinet is informed by the field-defining work of Mark Solms and Ariane Bazan and their respective Freudian or Lacanian origins. Asking questions on the relevance of neuropsychoanalysis in a clinical setting, this book offers vital insight into how analysts can bring this field into their day-to-day work with clients. Clinical and other interludes illustrate and illuminate the matter from the perspective of the psychoanalyst at work.

Written in an accessible style and part of The Routledge Neuropsychoanalysis Series, this volume will interest both those experienced with neuropsychoanalysis and those approaching the topic for the first time.

Mark Kinet is a psychiatrist, psychotherapist, and psychoanalyst. He has authored, or (co-)edited, some 30 books on psychiatry and psychotherapy, psychoanalysis, and culture issues. His website can be found at www.markkinet.be.

The Routledge Neuropsychoanalysis Series
Series editor: Mark Solms

The attempt to integrate the findings and methods of psychoanalysis with those of the neurological sciences can be said to have begun in 1895, with Freud's *Project for a Scientific Psychology*. Ongoing, sporadic efforts continued throughout the 20th century. However, the field really took off when the journal *Neuropsychoanalysis* was founded in 1999 and the International Neuropsychoanalysis Society was established in 2000. Ever since, a themed annual congress has been held in different cities around the world. Today, it is fair to say that these efforts have generated the most rapidly growing and influential body of knowledge and clinical practice in the broader field of psychoanalysis.

The establishment of this book series in 2023 marked another important milestone in the development of the field. Under the editorship of Mark Solms, the co-chair of the International Neuropsychoanalysis Society, it publishes books by leading proponents – and critics – of neuropsychoanalysis. The books in this series focus not only on the scientific findings of neuropsychoanalysis and on its theoretical yield, but also on its history, its philosophical implications and its clinical practice, as well as its ramifications for neighbouring disciplines and for the mental and neurological sciences as a whole.

Titles in this series include:

The Spirit of the Drive in Neuropsychoanalysis
Mark Kinet

For more information about this series, please visit https://www.routledge.com/The-Routledge-Neuropsychoanalysis-Series/book-series/RNS

The Spirit of the Drive in Neuropsychoanalysis

Mark Kinet

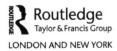

Routledge
Taylor & Francis Group

LONDON AND NEW YORK

Designed cover image: © Greet Desal, *Sleepers Peace*, 2017, acryl polyester, 105 x 90 x 35 cm.

First published in English 2024
by Routledge
4 Park Square, Milton Park, Abingdon, Oxon OX14 4RN

and by Routledge
605 Third Avenue, New York, NY 10158

Routledge is an imprint of the Taylor & Francis Group, an informa business

Published in Dutch by Gompel & Svacina 2022

British Library Cataloguing-in-Publication Data
A catalogue record for this book is available from the British Library

Library of Congress Cataloging-in-Publication Data
Names: Kinet, Mark, author.
Title: The spirit of the drive in neuropsychoanalysis / Mark Kinet.
Description: Abingdon, Oxon ; New York, NY : Routledge, 2024. |
Series: The Routledge neuropsychoanalysis series | Includes
bibliographical references and index. |
Identifiers: LCCN 2023025479 (print) | LCCN 2023025480 (ebook) |
ISBN 9781032495446 (paperback) | ISBN 9781032495484 (hardback) |
ISBN 9781003394358 (ebook)
Subjects: LCSH: Psychoanalysis. | Neurosciences. |
Neuropsychiatry. | Psychotherapy.
Classification: LCC RC506 .K524 2024 (print) | LCC RC506
(ebook) | DDC 616.89/17—dc23/eng/20230817
LC record available at https://lccn.loc.gov/2023025479
LC ebook record available at https://lccn.loc.gov/2023025480

ISBN: 978-1-032-49548-4 (hbk)
ISBN: 978-1-032-49544-6 (pbk)
ISBN: 978-1-003-39435-8 (ebk)

DOI: 10.4324/9781003394358

Typeset in Times New Roman
by codeMantra

Contents

Chapter 1

Prologue

Back then, my father and I would have endless fun at sports and games. What we liked to do, for instance, was a romp in the water with a ball. We were as happy as dolphins. We swam and dived to our hearts' content. We often enjoyed pushing the ball underwater as deep as we could for as long as possible. This took both energy and agility. Sooner or later, however, we would have to give in. The ball would finally escape our grasp and then sometimes jump metres high above the surface. It rarely, if ever, did this in a straight line and sometimes emerged far away next to us or behind us. The course it took underwater proved surprisingly more erratic than expected. It would often even happen that the ball would seem to reappear *as if out of nowhere*.

Some characteristics of Freud's dynamic unconscious can be deduced from such pleasurable scenes that took place sometimes on the North Sea, the lakes of Carinthia or the Albert Canal in Antwerp. First, certain things are pushed under the surface, and then what was repressed will return sooner or later. It is a mechanism underlying many seemingly puzzling psychological problems. First, we push content we need to figure out what to do with or don't like *out of* our awareness in all sorts of ways. Then, thoughts or feelings will take possession of us sooner or later without understanding where they come from. We experience fear, anger, agitation or sadness, but we cannot reach these emotions with reason or master them. We have a phobia of cats even though we know they can do little or nothing to harm us. We have cruel compulsions that constantly impose on us, even towards the most innocent creatures around us. We vent our frustrations at the wrong time or the wrong person. We feel deeply hurt or short-changed for a (perceived) slight. On closer inspection, our lives teem with moments when we say one thing and do another and yet another.

If undesirable matters continue to intrude, we must use additional means[1] to eliminate them. We must put more energy into 'domestic affairs' without realising it. This can compromise our psychic economy and sometimes even our 'foreign affairs'. Freud makes an apt comparison in this regard. According to him, our psyche gets weakened by inner conflict and, like a country in civil war, we need the support of an external ally.[2] Good advice, information and the power of our own or someone else's reason are primarily powerless against such phenomena. Something at

DOI: 10.4324/9781003394358-1

work within us is more potent than we are ourselves. We don't understand it, but it keeps its hold over us. We may even feel hopelessly trapped. We want to flee or *something* to change, but preferably without having to change *ourselves.*

Besides this dynamic or demonic unconscious that determines our life (experiences) like some Ego-alien force, you also have another (and more descriptive) unconscious. Virtually ninety-five percent of our mental activity is automatic and non-conscious. Strangely, this is not different for our perceptual and cognitive processes. We only know half of what we hear or see, and our cognitive faculties are constantly mobilised outside our knowledge or awareness. Our conscious mind, then, only has a minimal capacity. It is little more than a significant simplification that tries to guide us through everyday problems with, at most, seven to nine available bits of information (an international phone number, say). In a sense, we live on autopilot most of the time. In contemporary computer terms, we are guided by algorithms. We only deviate if we have to. When or as long as everything goes *according to plan,* we allow ourselves to be guided blindly by built-in drivers. We only 'wake up' when their predictions fail to materialise or lead us into difficulties, or we stumble over them.

I repeatedly use the following analogy in this context. We were taught to drive a car in a certain way. A breakdown or accident can happen to anyone. Still, something is wrong when we repeatedly have technical problems, run off the road, crash into a tree, incur fines for traffic violations or collide with other road users. We might do well to examine our vehicle or driving style closely. Hidden flaws are probably at the root of our recurring difficulties. Unless we get to the heart of the problem and tackle it, a lasting solution to the problem is unlikely to be found. Psychoanalysis then clarifies why and how all these unconscious factors continue to exert their shaping influence throughout our lives. They appear 'live on stage' to be understood and worked on within the therapeutic relationship.[3]

From a steadfast integrative mindset, I have always taken a broad and multicultural stance. This holds, too, for the psychoanalytic movement. According to Albert Rothenberg,[4] creativity involves the ability to imagine opposing ideas. Divergence (if not dissidence) would thus contribute to originality. Why (only) listen to like-minded people? Isn't it so that the most extraordinary richness can be found in encounters with strangers or unfamiliar things? Doesn't exogamy most often lead to children who flourish? The French have a nice expression for this: *Du choc des idées jaillit la lumière.* Ideas that collide make something light up. Regarding the depth and breadth of their thought, I consider Freud and Lacan the two greatest psychoanalytic thinkers.[5] Beyond them, I have found inspiration mainly from authors as diverse as Melanie Klein, Wilfred Bion, Donald Winnicott and Peter Fonagy. Paul Verhaeghe is probably the most influential theory teacher among my fellow Flemish speakers. He combines in an original way Freud, Lacan and Fonagy.[6]

While psychoanalysis is now about a hundred and twenty-five years old, this book is about a discipline which is only a young adult neuropsychoanalysis. As soon as I started working as a neuropsychiatrist, I was inquisitive about input from neuroscientific quarters. Of course, I am well aware of the Freudian dictum[7] that any progress is only half as significant as it initially appears. Yet, this interest

quickly grew into enthusiasm, thanks to the illuminating, evolving work of neuropsychoanalytic founder Mark Solms[8] and my compatriot Ariane Bazan.[9] The
former is a professor in Cape Town, the latter in Nancy and Brussels. I read all of
Solms's books and most of his articles. I also watched or listened to dozens of his
lectures which can be found on *YouTube*. Under the motto *learn while you move,*
I am generally a lover of audio recordings. I appreciate that they are suited to all
postures and many motor activities. They also have the character of private lessons.
You get to know the speakers almost personally. They share scientific knowledge
and experience spontaneously and colloquially. Each voice has a different tone
or timbre. The added pleasure of tics, anecdotes or witticisms makes this form of
knowledge transfer resemble a Spielbergian *Close encounter of the fourth kind.*

I tried meeting Mark Solms at the beautiful Belmond Mount Nelson Hotel in
Cape Town while visiting South Africa. Still, he informed me that at that time,
he was in the United Kingdom and the United States by invitation. I had been
in personal contact with Ariane Bazan on several occasions. We edited a book
together in 2010 entitled *Psychoanalysis and Neuroscience,*[10] and she had also
written remarkable and noteworthy neuropsychoanalytic contributions to other
books I edited.

To be clear, I am neither an academic nor a neuropsychoanalyst. I have, however,
been working full-time clinically for over thirty years: as a psychiatrist in a (semi-)
residential psychotherapeutic setting and in an independent outpatient psychoanalytic practice. I am more inclined to pragmatism than to dogmatism. As a pun,
my way of thinking might be called *paradigmatic*. I have authored or (co-)edited
over thirty books on the most diverse topics related to psychiatry, psychotherapy,
psychoanalysis and culture. I have also followed with unfailing interest as many
new scientific and societal developments as possible. With an educational background in natural sciences and humanities, I have always been interested in their
cross-fertilisation. It sometimes produces tasty fruit that is also rich in vitamins.

This is particularly true of the research findings within the (still fledgling)
neurosciences. I was initially amused mainly by specific correlations and analogies
between these findings and my experience in the clinic. There are the little things.
For instance, in the homunculus on somatosensory and motor brain/Penfield
maps,[11] the feet appear next to the sex organs. A neuroscientific 'explanation' for
foot fetishism? Or consider another example: (electrical) stimulation of rats' *nucleus accumbens* (the 'pleasure nucleus') appears to take precedence over their
survival instinct.[12] Is this 'evidence' for Lacan's enjoyment/*jouissance,* which
leads beyond the pleasure principle? But more extensive insights also piqued my
interest. After all, our brains appeared to be teeming with dynamic forces colli-
ding. First, the brain works at two speeds: the slower, higher functions versus the
faster (epi-)limbic ones. There is a phenomenon of lateralisation at play between
the hemispheres: the left hemisphere is more rational and inhibitory, the right more
irrational and holistic.[13] Information mainly excites the left hemisphere and emotions the right.[14] The inhibitory/regulatory role of the Ego has long been associated
with that of the prefrontal cortex. This is compatible with Freud's model of the primary process as the carrier of content and the secondary process as the admission

condition for consciousness.[15] Last but not least, we have known since Paul MacLean's theory of the triune brain[16] that there is also, for palaeontological reasons, a vessel of contradictions under our skull.

An earlier Dutch version of this book appeared in 2022 as the 32nd in the series *Psychoanalytisch Actueel* (Current Psychoanalytics), of which I am the editor-in-chief. The present book is an updated version, elaborated and translated into English.[17] It attempts to report on what appeals to me in neuropsychoanalysis and why. In particular, I pay attention to developments that could be genuinely inspiring in wider intellectual circles. I explain and comment on this complex subject matter in the simplest terms possible. This information is based on many hundreds of neuroscientific studies and experiments, all highly technical and specialised. Therefore, within this scope, I can only present the conclusions that can be drawn from them. To keep a smooth reading of the book, I refer to this specialised work where necessary in notes and extensive references at the back of the book. To illustrate the subject matter but also to enlighten and entertain, I have provided the reader with more playful interludes from time to time. Both life experience and my broader psychoanalytic activity shine through these asides. They are testimony of the precisely human 'cortico-thalamic capacity for satisfying their needs in imaginary and symbolic ways'.[18]

In these interludes, I have tried (only to a limited extent, of course) to put into practice instructions from Vladimir Nabokov in his *Lectures on Literature*. There he sets the writer a triple task: story-teller, teacher and ... enchanter.[19] The latter is as important to me as the first two. Paradoxically, the dirtiest part of the body is the mind. It may even be our most important erogenous zone! So what do I wish the reader above all? Enjoyment! We shall see that it's the *feel* of the drive.

Endnotes

1 We can use psychic mechanisms as 'means' (Anna Freud's [1936] defence mechanisms). Still, we can also use various external means (work, sex, alcohol, drugs, food, shopping and so on) to 'get rid' of difficult feelings and obtain a 'good' feeling; at the same time, narcotics are usually pleasure/enjoyment products too. For a more recent overview of (different levels of) defence mechanisms, see Vaillant (1995).
2 Freud (1940a, p. 471; 1940b, p. 172).
3 On how they come *live on stage*, see Kinet (2022c) recently.
4 Rothenberg (1971).
5 They cover the entire breadth of psychology and psychopathology: neurosis, psychosis *and* perversion; they investigate individual and cultural phenomena, developmental psychology, sexuality and aggression, drive, object, self, etc. From the beginning, I will stress that Freud and Lacan lived in different contexts and eras. Freud had his roots in the natural sciences of the Helmholtz School of Physiology and entered the psychiatry field via hypnosis and hysteria. Lacan borrowed materials from three disciplines, enabling him to build his theoretical edifice. From developmental psychology (and in particular the work of Henri Wallon on the formation of identity in the child), he borrowed the mirror stage; from anthropology, and in particular the work of Claude Lévi-Strauss, he borrowed the distinction between real, imaginary and symbolic; and

from structural linguistics, and in particular the work of Ferdinand de Saussure, the contrast that the linguist makes between signifier and signified. He wrote his doctoral thesis on paranoid psychosis. Sometimes, Lacan's desire to build a deductive metapsychological theory implies a controversial tendency towards abstraction and speculative theorisation. For some, it seems more based on a system of thought than on rigorous observation of mental suffering and dysfunction. *Quod non*, however. In *Pour l'amour de Lacan*, Derrida (1980) lauds Lacan's philosophical sophistication. On the other hand, Lacan always stresses that the difference between his thought and that of the philosopher is that his thinking is firmly grounded in his practice/the clinical situation (Mooij 2002, p. 30).

6 Paul Verhaeghe was awarded the Goethe prize by the *Canadian Psychological Association* in 2004 for his *On being normal and other disorders*. Award winners like Nancy McWilliams, Peter Fonagy, Ansermet and Magistretti, Patrick Luyten and Charles Strozier are referred to elsewhere in this book.

7 Quote of Nestroy in Freud (1926c, p. 289; 1926d, p. 197).

8 For Solms' C. V. and publications, see https://www.ipu-berlin.de/fileadmin/profile/curriculum-vitae/solms-cv.pdf

9 For Bazan's C. V. and publications, see http://www.arianebazan.be/wp-content/uploads/2013/04/CV_Ariane_Bazan_Ao%C3%BBt_2021-site.pdf

10 Kinet and Bazan (2010).

11 Penfield and Boldrey (1937).

12 Olds and Milner (1954).

13 De Kroon (2005, p. 146).

14 Leffert (2010, p. 106).

15 Bazan (2007a, 2011b).

16 In the 1960s, the idea was that a reptilian brain (*basal ganglia*), an ancient mammalian brain (limbic system) and a more recent mammalian brain (neocortex) emerged successively and with their operating principles on top of each other throughout our natural history. Respectively, they determine our drives, instincts and rational thinking (MacLean 1990).

17 According to Robert Frost, poetry is what gets lost in translation. I did my best to avoid this loss of 'poetry' as much as possible.

18 Solms (2018b, p. 5).

19 Nabokov (1980).

Chapter 2

Interlude

Das Hundbewusste

It is no criticism of the British way of life, Martin (son of Sigmund) Freud wrote, to suggest that a British family dog appears to be the essential member of the family.[1] However, this is not a British prerogative because Freud's Austrian family was very keen on dogs too. Sigmund Freud had a Chinese chow, and his daughter Anna had a German shepherd. They both barked vigorously at each patient who entered the Berggasse, but Jofi, the chow, was so well trained that she was often present during Freud's psychoanalytic sessions. Thanks to Jofi's internal clock, her master didn't need a watch to end the consultation on time.[2]

Roy Grinker's account of his analysis with Freud is very telling in this regard.[3] Once, when he was very emotional, Jofi jumped on top of him, and Freud said: You see, Jofi is so excited that you've discovered the source of your anxiety![4] Yofi means beautiful in Hebrew, and it seems she had exquisite psychoanalytic sensibilities.[5] But this is rather exceptional, especially compared to our limited experience.

We have had a black Labrador in our midst for several years now. His name is Bruce. Not Springsteen, Lee or Willis but Almighty. He was born in a litter of eleven. We started visiting him during the first few weeks of his life. His mother barely ate anything. She sacrificed herself during day and night shifts to serve half her offspring. She was utterly knackered. I wonder why we chose Bruce in particular. According to the breeder, he was the calmest of the litter. It makes us wonder how the other pups developed ...

Bruce has an impressive pedigree with his working line.[6] His father was a champion of England. We saw a picture of him with his tail stretched, looking at a point beyond the horizon as if he were on Newfoundland's coast. Meanwhile, one of his brothers is emerging as a prize rescuer in the Swiss Alps. So my wife bought Bruce a red leather collar with white crosses. He looks super-reliable in it – *Quod non*, of course.

We think Bruce is the sweetest and most handsome dog in the world. He is aero-dynamic, like a shiny bullet. Sometimes black angel, sometimes black devil, he is our eternal baby. Our life gradually became completely organised around his creature comforts. His passive vocabulary has now grown to some fifty terms. He does

DOI: 10.4324/9781003394358-2

not care about semantics and grammar but immediately recognises the so-called motherese of sounds, tone and timbre.

Many dogs resemble their master. Like our car, Bruce would reflect a piece of us or, like a child, he would inherit parental narcissism. He is our beloved if not idealised, alter-ego. In addition, he loves us unconditionally and accepts us completely. He understands us without words yet knows how to attune to our talks with body language. He has something of the all-good mother who gives and grants us everything on both good and bad days. Sometimes, he watches over us or takes care of us. Then, he is a cross between bodyguard and guardian angel or more precisely: janitor. He embodies an archaic parental image in every way while we feel like the royalty he is so eager to please.

We can also learn a lot from him about different aspects of our unconscious. Our species have been mammals for two hundred and fifty million years and have a large piece of our brain in common. Significantly, we differ in terms of the prefrontal cortex. Both in volume and connectivity, this cortex is proportionally much more significant in humans. It produces inhibition, enables thinking and ensures we are mainly ignorant of our true motivations. The ability to think symbolically, our theory of mind, and mental time travel are neo-cortical attributes.[7]

Genetically, the difference between humans and bonobos is no more significant than between the Indian and African elephants. Our intellectual abilities are incomparable, but they are morally neutral. One can do much good as well as harm with intelligence. Our ethical concerns, on the one hand, extend to things and creates different (even radically different) from us. On the other hand, we succeed like no other animal in harming the other-similar, starting with our (mother) nature. Fortunately, there is an eloquent word for it: the Anthropocene.

Affective neuroscientists explicitly distinguish between drive and instinct. The former resides high in the brain stem. There pleasure and unpleasure are the compasses by which inner/homeostatic processes are evaluated. The drive is classically the measure of the work demanded of our soul life: to restore disturbed equilibria (unpleasure) by restored balances (pleasure). Instincts are higher up in the limbic system. They involve fixed modes of behaviour and reaction patterns, including emotional ones, in dealing with the environment. The migration of birds, salmon swimming upstream, the hibernation of bears: these actions do not need not be learned but are evolutionarily pre-wired. The consensus today is that humans share several emotional-instinctive systems with all mammals. They are written below in capitals because they relate to anatomic-physiologically distinct circuits common to all mammals. I'll let Bruce illustrate them briefly.

First and foremost, there is the SEEKING or WANTING system. Bruce begins an enthusiastic and wagging exploration of the environment when he gets outside. He takes pleasure in searching/hunting for new stimuli or treasures.

The LIKING system complements this system. Sometimes, Bruce finds something he likes or that satisfies his desires. This produces a certain satisfaction, and henceforth, he knows precisely where to find 'it'. Things can get complicated, however. What if his hunger is short-circuited by his favourite boss arriving home from work? Is an urge to pee driving him into the garden, or is he into play? At times, he has a 'mind in conflict'![8]

Then, there is the LUST system. When Bruce encounters a female, he immediately senses her. Beyond this, his love remains rather courtly. Possibly due to the culture in which he grew up. He never humps our legs, even though the slightest pleasure immediately produces blood-coloured evidence of his excitement.

Then, there is the FEAR-AVOIDANCE system. Bruce doesn't have to learn that you shouldn't jump down stairs or from other heights. His predecessors who took this risk did not survive the evolutionary process: a hard fact that also does not facilitate reproduction.

Then there is the RAGE system: if Bruce is cornered or another creature predatorily targets him, he barks or snaps. The enemy must be destroyed. This is a form of hot aggression to be distinguished from the cold-bloodedness that characterises the predator pursuing its prey. Inter-male aggression is a sub-variant. Bruce bites the flank of his opponents, or he stands with much swagger and loud barking 'on his mark', but he will not do more harm, nor does he engage in a fight.

The ATTACHMENT system is (adaptively) essential to any mammal. In distress, it calls 'mum' on whose care it depends, after all, for survival. In the first months of baby Bruce's life, we did not need a baby monitor to provide timely care for his needs. If the 'caretaker' stays away too long, the 'youngster' falls silent. That way, he does not needlessly waste energy, remains close to the home environment and easily avoids becoming a victim because he is without defence. Yes, nature is ingenious indeed.

The inverse of the ATTACHMENT system is the CARE system. Confrontation with life in distress mobilises a caring and protective reflex. To the regret of those who envy it, the females of a species of mammals are evolutionarily better equipped to mobilise both instinctive patterns. Bruce found a little hedgehog caught dorsally among the rose bushes. Carefully he freed it from this thorny position. I don't know if this detracts from his masculinity.

Last but not least, there is a PLAY system. All mammals have some play drive. If mice have not had their playtime one day, they have to make up for the loss with an extra half hour the next day. While playing (with some necessary bruises), they learn all sorts of things in terms of (also social) skills and limitations. Bruce puts his front paws on the ground, wags his hindquarters and invites us into the game (Latin: *in lusio*) at appropriate times.

Paraphrasing German writer Juli Zeh[9]: If everything is playing, we are lost; if not, we are lost, definitely.

Endnotes

1 Freud (1973, p. 379).
2 Beck (2010).
3 Grinker (2001).

4 See http://www.virtualpsychoanalyticmuseum.org/wp-content/uploads/2017/10/ Beneveniste-on-Sigmund-Freud-and-His-Love-of-Dogs.pdf

5 In his 1961–1962 Seminar on identification, Jacques Lacan (2002) points at his dog Justine to mark the difference between the pre-verbal and the verbal. Justine has speech but not language. Insofar as she speaks, she is not capable of transference, and she lives only in the 'demand'. See later in this book.

6 The most crucial purpose of the working line is for the dog to bring game that has been shot back to its owner.

7 In this interlude, I skip the (neuro-)biological references, but this will be abundantly compensated later.

8 I refer to a psychoanalytic classic: *The Mind in Conflict*, Brenner (1982).

9 Zeh (2007).

Chapter 3

A Vase or the Two Faces

Neuropsy

Until the 1980s, a doctor specialising as a neuropsychiatrist in our area had to train in neurology and psychiatry. The relationship between these two fields determined their final professional profile. Today, most psychiatrists and neurologists know little about each other's fields. More generally, there is also a sharp divide between the two, scientifically and socially. These fields share this fate with psychoanalysis versus neuroscience or psychiatry.[1] Thus, in Rubin's[2] optical illusion, one can never simultaneously see the two faces and the vase. Nevertheless, we must maintain, willy-nilly, both perspectives to acquire the entire possible picture of our thinking and feeling.[3] To a clinician like me, whether you call this the split between the natural sciences and the humanities, dual aspect (but ontological) monism or epistemological dualism[4] is a matter for scholastic philosophers. Reportedly, these philosophers are said never to have agreed on the genus of angels.

That lightning and thunder reach different senses at different times is a fact. They come – *dixit* Solms – from the same source, but neither is the other's cause, nor can you reduce the one to the other.[5] Even more dialectically, by the way, a reduction is to be discouraged. You can examine bodies physically, chemically or biologically. Laws from a previous level remain unaffected but are supplemented by others that only apply to this higher level and only do justice to their respective idiosyncrasies. Specifically *human*, every science is faced with a double task. It consists of explaining, understanding, counting, recounting, quantifying and deciphering.[6] Even for psychoanalysis as a science, it is often (as for Odysseus) navigating between two whirlpools: the Scylla of free association (on the sofa or not) in the consulting room and the Charybdis of empirical research in the various manifestations of the lab.[7] Finally, I might remind the reader of what a character in one of the novels by Dutch author Harry Mulisch once said: 'The world is a soup, and our thinking is a fork!'[8]

After two decades of research, South African neuropsychologist and psychoanalyst Mark Solms christened neuropsychoanalysis (and its journal) as a discipline in its own right in 1999. The founding conference of the *International Neuropsychoanalysis Society* took place in 2000 and was chaired by him.[9] Nobel laureate Eric Kandel has become the best-known advocate of this neuropsychoanalysis since his *The Age of Insight*.[10] Even before its birth, he assigned the combination of

DOI: 10.4324/9781003394358-3

neuroscience and psychoanalysis the role of the *New intellectual framework for psychiatry*.[11] Since then, neuropsychoanalysis has contributed much to psychoanalytic insights on memory, drive, dreams, the structural (Id/Ego/Superego) model and the dynamic unconscious.[12] Correlating ideographic clinical practice and nomothetic research clarifies theory, strengthens a more (natural) scientific basis for psychoanalysis, restores the social prestige it lost after the Second World War[13] and inspires therapeutic practice. One of the primary endeavours of neuropsychoanalysis is to avoid needless neurosimplifications and reductions.

Classically, unconscious processes are *the* object of psychoanalytic research. You cannot observe them directly more than examining darkness with a torch.[14] We must make do with the *unconscious formations*[15] such as the dream, the symptom, parapraxes, transference[16] or acting out. These can only be adequately understood through the hypothesis of the unconscious. This is why I like to call psychoanalysis the science of traces. Like a detective, it primarily has to make do with *circumstantial evidence*. But you can also call it the science of the unreasonable. I am reminded of Lord Polonius' words from Hamlet: *Though this be madness, yet there is method in 't*.[17] For madness, too, has its reason. According to Jacques Lacan, psychoanalysis was, above all, *science du particulier*[18]: the science of the *particular*. It investigates laws that only apply at $n = 1$. This $n = 1$ is not so much the physical uniqueness of fingerprint, retina or DNA. Instead, it is the singularity through which we, as subjects, constantly say and write ourselves and thus make something new or our own of our history.[19] In this context, I would like to refer to an elegant formulation by Vincent de Gaulejac: '*L'homme est le produit d'une histoire dont il cherche à devenir le sujet*'. Man is the product of a history of which he tries to become the subject.[20]

For a long time, behavioural observations (e.g. in *infant research*) were considered inappropriate for psychoanalysis.[21] They were from outside the consulting room and therefore remained controversial. While subjective and hermeneutic–empathic analysis is hypothesis-generating like no other, the empirical and third-person research perspective (which also characterises neuroscience) can produce hypothesis-confirming correlations.[22] Wasn't Adolf Grünbaum's philosophical critique of science[23] precisely that psychoanalysis needs empirical support *independent* of its clinical context? If not, its ubiquitous circular reasoning remains pernicious for its scientific credit.[24] Yet, to Solms, the clinical situation remains a last court of appeal. In this, therefore, he is not so far from Lacan with his statement: '*La psychanalyse n'a qu'un medium: la parole du patient*'.[25] Psychoanalysis has only one medium: the patient's speech.

Science Fiction

Classical science, in pursuit of objectivity, seeks to exclude the subjective/subject. Psychoanalysis as a science of the subject eminently undermines this scientific premise. After all, it is not only a science of or about the subjective and the unconscious but paradoxically has its basis there.[26] We know Freud's grandiose comparison, calling the introduction of his unconscious a third affront after those of Copernicus and Darwin. The findings of the latter two have since become commonplace, while the unconscious remains controversial. Probably because the unconscious undermines the consistency of knowing *itself*. Jacques Lacan, therefore, speaks of *subversion* (rather than revolution) concerning psychoanalysis.[27] To psychoanalysis, the Cartesian *cogito* that supports our (in this case, scientific) imagination is a product of our imagination. For it, every practice of science is, in this double sense a form of science fiction.

Now, Lacan has a tenacious reputation for being clinically irrelevant. Nevertheless, his distinction between the real, imaginary and symbolic order can provide a valuable and overarching frame of reference for the so-called and widely used biopsychosocial model.[28] In a Lacanian view, all that is human from our primaeval times have become inextricably intertwined. Indeed, the unmentionable *Schmerz* of the *infans*[29] presupposes a specific answer from the big Other based on which the subject begins its historiography.[30] I use the real here (somewhat differently from Lacan) as the real of natural science. For example, the real as the energetic-material but also as other Things such as disposition, drive, trauma or (modern) arousal, as many attempts to grasp this real in concepts.[31] As early as Galileo Galilei, mathematics was the language of nature. Einstein's famous $E = mc^2$ illustrates this. The latter also comes with the motto that we should make things as simple as possible … but not simpler. Later, in this book, we will see how successful Mark Solms is at doing this with a kind of razor of Ockham.[32]

Secondly, after the real, there is the imaginary of attachment and seduction we share with the animals. As elaborated later, it is also the register of the mirror and the other-similar of imagination and misunderstanding. Finally, there is the specifically human, namely the symbolic of language and lack, of law and history.[33] I refer for a moment to the clinic. Every psychiatrist or therapist knows and experiences every day that treatment works through three possible angles of approach that are classically used simultaneously or consecutively in a sophisticated and balanced combination. There is the biological influence, which acts on the real. The therapeutic (confidential and trust) relationship operates on attachment. Based on this kind of 'work', mental and emotional development is facilitated. Finally, there is the (life-) history within which signifiers (also in the form of the here-and-now of transference) resonate. The psychiatrist's vehicles are the natural sciences and the humanities. Some call this uncomfortable position a *grand écart*.[34] By all means, signs and meaning apply in psychiatry, explaining and understanding, cause and coherence.[35]

The knowledge that psychiatry develops about the particular case refers, on the one hand, to general laws insofar as it is the clinic of the sign (of the disease). Appendicitis has similar symptoms Everywhere and Always because it is characterised by natural causality. Here, the substrate is the somatic-physical underlying psycho-(patho)-logy. On the other hand, it refers to the clinic of the signifier, which we will see refers only to other signifiers.[36] Diachronously to signifiers from life history and synchronously to signifiers from the transference–countertransference continuum that unfolds between patient and therapist. Moreover, psychic causality with its particularity, disproportion, circular and *nachträgliche*/deferred action or afterwardsness causality applies.[37] This asymmetry between explaining and understanding is sometimes called the central and foundational *manco* of psychiatry (and of the subject).[38]

In Search of Lost Mind

However, this manco or lack is repeatedly denied or repressed. In the process, psychiatry seemingly *loses its mind*. In its pursuit of objectivity, the (inter-)subjectivity that precisely characterises the relationship between patient and therapist is lost. There is a danger of a sometimes alarming impoverishment of the clinical encounter. Ahistorism[39] and decontextualisation[40] become trumps. The technification and medicalisation of happiness arise with an overestimation of the impact of the rational. The therapist knows (it is supposed) what is normal/expected and abnormal, as well as the (shortest and fastest) way to happiness and pleasure. He 'cures' the patient's 'ignorance', and thus the path to both is paved. In other words, there is a naive belief in the therapeutic efficacy of knowledge.

The illusion is created today (by selling a nineteenth-century view [*Geisteskrankheiten sind Gehirnkrankheiten* – dixit Wilhelm Griesinger] as old wine in new bottles); all mental suffering belongs to the domain of medicine. Now, everyone is excited about medical science's scientific and technological advances. Whether or not fitted with new joints, blood vessels or other parts, someone's life expectancy and quality of life have increased in the (mainly Western) world. Psychiatry has also participated in these developments. Since the 1950s and 1960s, psychopharmaceuticals have emerged for major psychiatric disorders (depression, mania, schizophrenia and so on). Their efficacy has been scientifically proven. The quality of life of millions of psychiatric patients has increased significantly, thanks to the judicious use of these drugs. Meanwhile, however, all these drugs have created expectations that seem to be certainties. Their prescription would end the patient's suffering and do so *'cito, tuto et iucunde'*: quickly, effectively and with minimal inconvenience. Above all, the patient no longer needs to commit. There is an 'external' peg on which to hang his difficulties. It is the famous exteriorising inherent in the Kleinian schizoid–paranoid position. The 'evil' is thus split off and projected outwards rather than situated internally.[41]

Meanwhile, one of the pillars of psychiatry (the humanities) is in danger of finally dying under (neuro-)biological reductionism. In this process, a complete explanation would make understanding superfluous. This view assumes that the connection between psychological and physical phenomena can ultimately be understood. Biomedical sciences are placed above the humanities, empiricism above hermeneutics and quantitative above qualitative research. One consequence is that internal research validity and efficacy precede ecological validity and effectiveness. And this, while psychiatry (cf above) requires the complementarity of different levels of explanation, each with its methodology and epistemology.[42] Psychologies that explain and psychologies that understand are not mutually exclusive but overlap. However, it should be stated that explanatory or objective psychology paradoxically leads to a psychology without a psyche.[43] We recall what the famous neurologist Oliver Sacks[44] said: 'Neuropsychology is admirable, but it excludes the psyche'.

The last century ended with 'the decade of the brain'. Neuroscience made great leaps forward. It can finally be shown that the structure, as well as the function of the brain, is influenced by environmental factors. Thanks to various techniques – such as positron emission tomography (PET), functional magnetic resonance imaging (fMRI) and event-related potential (ERP) – it is now possible to visualise not only the anatomy but also the functioning of the brain. The advantage is that the (by definition, hidden or invisible) world of the psyche, thoughts, feelings and fantasies can be made visible and tangible. Psychiatry can, at last, sit at the table with its big brothers in the natural sciences and participate in discussions about *real* and *serious* matters. After all, medicine has traditionally treated the psyche/invisible as its poor relation. In its view, what transcends the visible is often unreal.[45]

Most mental problems can indeed not be *seen*. Moreover, most psychologically suffering patients do not allow themselves to be cared for but try to hide. As such, they are a priori problematic for medicine. Characterised as it is by the clinic of the gaze, medicine only 'believes' what can be made visible in numbers (lab), by imaging or based on all kinds of glass fibres that can penetrate various orifices of the body. Not only concerning psycho-trauma and psychological problems (and psychotherapy) in general, there are believers and non-believers. The latter are like the unbelieving Thomas, who wants to witness Christ's stigmata with his own eyes. With its motion pictures, neuroimaging manages to convince these non-believers of the existence of psychic realities. The influence of environment and therapy can also finally be made visible.[46] According to many neuropsychology critics, this increase in visual knowledge leads to localising psychic activity but not understanding it. Not *that* psychological problems correlate to a neurological substrate/process, but *how and why* they do so remained the most challenging question in the brain–mind dilemma.[47]

Controversial?

Either way, the relationship between psychoanalysis and neuroscience remains controversial. To his fellow neuroscientists, Solms' psychoanalytic *démarche* was like an astronomer suddenly turning to astrology. Mark Solms and Oliver Turnbull[48] experienced it first-hand: psychoanalytic interest leads to a loss of respect from colleagues, student appreciation and an unwillingness of academic journals to publish work inspired by this field. With psychoanalysis, it is, at any rate, challenging to advance.[49] Combining it with neuroscience is downright 'bad for your career'.[50]

However, the resistance of the psychoanalytic world towards neuroscience was even more significant. Blass and Carmeli,[51] for example, were and remain[52] downright hostile. Indeed, they see the influence of neuroscience as a threat to *proper* psychoanalysis.[53] They are a model of those to whom the prefix *neuro-* signifies the reduction of the psychic to the measurable. Neurosis, in this view, is reduced to disturbed brain functioning, and there is a risk of patients asking questions about their brains rather than themselves. For them, neuro-language functions as a meta-language that is supposed to enrich all mind disciplines through an omniscient discourse because neuro-know-how would grasp how the brain or mind works.[54] Neuropsychoanalyst *avant-la-lettre* Howard Shevrin[55] already referred to prag-matic philosopher W. V. O. Quine when he stated that science is impossible without a quantifiable energy concept. However, many psychoanalysts hate numbers. As if using them would necessarily have a de-subjectifying effect on everything human. A statement by Paul Verhaeghe[56] is exemplary in this context: 'God is dead, but we bow to numbers'.

Mark Solms repeatedly points out that the allergy to the quantifiable is far removed from Freud. I quote Freud's initial ambition: to furnish a psychology that shall be a natural science: to represent psychical processes as quantitatively determinate states of specifiable material particles, thus making those processes perspicuous and free from contradiction.[57] Or, to put this aversion further into perspective: does the fact that it is made up of zeros and ones detract from the beauty of a CD on which Bach's St Matthew Passion is played? Lacanians, in particular, often have grave reservations about neuroscience. After all, the know-ledge on which psychoanalysis focusses, according to them, is '*un savoir insu à lui-même*'[58]: a knowledge unaware of itself. It is an unknowing knowing that resides (only) in the person's unconscious. What other sciences (especially the natural) know can be transmitted and is quantifiable, but – so they perhaps put it somewhat starkly – this unknowing knowing cannot be (re)counted, and any attempt at quantification fails.

Even in my Dutch-language area, many have strong reservations.[59] Others, in turn, have a more inclusive attitude towards neuroscientific views and findings.[60] Possibly this divergence of attitudes has to do with the difference between the *International Psychoanalytical Association* and the *Association Mondiale de Psychanalyse*,[61] between Anglo-Saxon and Roman culture,[62] between the empiri-cism of *I see* and the rationalism of *je comprends* (exemplified by Solms and Lacan, respectively), between the empirical and the hermeneutic approach or finally between analytic and continental philosophy. These are different positions regar-ding the dispersal to which all human sciences are by definition condemned and against which they each define their role.[63]

Patrick Luyten[64] wonders whether psychoanalysis is not guilty of *cherry-picking*. This involves the so-called *confirmation bias*: findings that suit them are eagerly cited. They significantly boost psychoanalysis's scientific *seriousness* and con-vince non-believers by making evidence visible. For his part, Paul Verhaeghe[65] suspects psychoanalysis of *physics envy*: a mocking pun, which he borrows from evolutionary psychologist Stephen Jay Gould.[66] So does psychoanalysis (or, even more broadly, psychiatry) want to sell its soul to that diabolical brain? The presence of neuroscientific references has been fully shown to increase scientific credibility significantly.[67] It is said that doctors get rich by translating words into Latin.

A patient comes to consult with a headache. Diagnosis: *cephalea*! (Latin for head-ache). Would neuroscience only translate psychoanalytic gibberish into more prestigious parlance?

Initially, I was also among the sceptics concerning the *Enthusiasm for the Brain*.[68] First and foremost, I was a fan of painters like Henri Matisse and Paul Gauguin. That's why I bumped into some of their quotes on the Internet. Matisse: '*L'exactitude n'est pas la vérité*'. The exact is not the truth. Gauguin: '*Je ferme les yeux pour voir*'. I close my eyes to see. Intuitively, I perceived man as at once a natural and biological but also a symbolic and sacred being. I saw the animal as one and man as two with nature. Even primates do not produce art, science or prayer. Nothing indicates that they are aware of the deathbed's specific human, future-perfect time. There is no symbolic language or order for them, as it is represented by the (law of the) father. By entering into the symbolic, an immediate naturalness is lost. Thus, there is a rupture with the biological, with man losing a piece of it (including of himself), as it were. In a Lacanian view, object small a is the rest of this loss, and as such, it acts as an object-cause of desire. It drives man towards some form of 'healing' and a supposedly original but – in fact – mythical enjoyment that can be harmful if not deadly. In Lacanian terms, it installs the human lack of being, his *manque-à-être*[69] or his want-to-be.[70]

Both in phylogenetic (*hominisation*) and ontogenetic development (*humanisation*), there needs to be a link as a logical (as opposed to chronological) rupture in this view.[71] The result is the anthropological difference that many psychiatrists and *a fortiori* (Lacanian) psychoanalysts insist on.[72] Psychiatry is a sub-specialisation of medicine, and the latter is considered an applied natural science. But human medicine is not veterinary.[73] They share an everyday biological and ethological basis but superimposed on this is the spiritual and cultural that denatures this dual basis. Our natural history remains operative but almost completely outstripped by our (micro- and macro-) *cultural* history.

I also wondered what the brain would have to tell us about the subjective subtleties and complexities of the consulting room. I shuddered at the tidal wave of neuro-essentialism.[74] With titles such as *We are our Brain*[75] or *L'homme Neuronal*,[76] it threatened to reduce our mental life to the workings of our grey cells. I was steeped in the prevailing model from the twentieth-century humanities without realising it sufficiently. They emphasised a social constructivist perspective: man as a self-creating cultural being. There, it was assumed that neuro- and evolutionary biology could teach us little or nothing about human nature. Man was, à la Nietzsche, the sick but also '*nicht festgestellte Tier*'.[77] He is fundamentally free – a *part of* but also *apart from nature.*

But aren't such views illustrative of a kind of humanistic hubris? I mentioned human narcissism/speciesism in another context, within which homo sapiens still dared to imagine themselves as the pinnacle of creation.[78] The Anthropocene (or is it à la philosopher of science Donna Haraway[79] more correctly: Capitalocene?) should have changed his mind by now. Perhaps the most universal/collective (delusional) human idea is that he is unique.

Universal and Unique

Paraphrasing Ryszard Kapuscinski,[80] world traveller and 'reporter of the century', every human being we meet anywhere in the world consists, as it were, of two beings; he is a duality that is difficult to split, something we are not always correctly aware of. One being is our spitting image: a human being with his joys and sorrows, his good days and bad days, who is happy with his successes, who does not like to be hungry, who does not want to be cold, who experiences pain as suffering and unhappiness and prosperity as satisfaction and fulfilment. The second being, overlying and intertwined with the first, is man as the bearer of culture, faith and beliefs. Neither being occurs in a pure and isolated state; they coexist and influence each other.

Translated to the matter at hand, the structure and functioning of our mind and brain are universal and conform to nomothetic or natural scientific laws. On the other hand, in humans, a vast neo-cortical cloak got pushed on top of our limbic system/emotional brain. We will see that this has created a largely unconscious medium between inside and outside. It is the unconscious as the long-sought *missing link* between the physical and the mental that Freud talks about in his letter to Georg Groddeck on 5 June 1917.[81] It is also Lacan's unconscious as the discourse of the big Other[82]: the meaning-generating structure that places itself between perception and consciousness. It forms, as it were, an invisible lens through which we see 'reality' and try to make something of it. It is linguistically structured and, in Lacan's famous formulation, is situated, as it were, between skin and flesh (*'entre cuir et chair'*).[83] The starting point here is our body, around which layers of meaning are draped.[84] The neo-cortical cloak moulds our identity by symbolically and imaginatively dressing a biological core. Our body is a limiting factor in this. It lays down the chalk lines. How they are filled in depends on the web of signifiers woven and written for and by us.[85] Thus, the treasury (Jacques Lacan: 'of the signifier') is gradually constituted according to the African proverb: every person who dies is a library that burns down.

This library is full of experiences and opinions. Our own and others. Many of its books also contain commandments and prohibitions, norms and values that interpret the ruling opinion or the opinion of those who rule. According to Paul Verhaeghe,[86] our identity is determined mainly by four relationships. Our relationship towards gender difference, towards elders and authorities, towards our other-similars and finally, our relationship with our body and ourselves. I am reminded of a famous poem by the Dutch poet H. H. Ter Balkt. It is titled *The Animal Crusade*. It portrays a rebellious trek of free-spirited animals who don't need to care about law, religion or morals and are happily travelling into the wild.[87] His verses illustrate the fullness of animals, which humans can sometimes look (not down on but) up to with envy, admiration or fear. I think of the primal power of the bison in prehistoric caves, of the fabulous animals of primitive religions or the horse of Freud's little Hans.[88]

While animals behave broadly the same way throughout the most widely separated centuries and places, humans are much more characterised by a dual cultural historicity. This comes from the big Other of civilisation and the big Other of education. How different is life in the twenty-first century from the fourteenth century in the Congo and Belgium? How different an upbringing can be even on the same High Street! There are at least two critical reasons for exceptional human historicity. First, we have the typically human neoteny. Evolution determined that at birth, there is a characteristic physiological immaturity and a prolonged helpless dependence of the new-born human child (biped position restricted pelvis' size precluded labour after the fortieth week of pregnancy and the process of [neuro-] development must continue and complete in an extrauterine environment). Furthermore, there is the fact that – in a way – the child is made of language and stories (or thrown into it). These factors create a well-nigh categorical rather than a gradual anthropological difference with our animal brothers and sisters.

Outlook

With all this as a *mindset,* I edited a book with my compatriot, Ariane Bazan, titled *Psychoanalysis and Neuroscience* in 2010. In a subsequent chapter, I reiterate my contribution to our brain's (experience-dependent and experience-independent) neuroplasticity.[89] It is most significant during childhood and adolescence but also remains active further in our lives (e.g. as a result of psychotherapy).[90] I also reiterate the different forms of memory(-circuits), each with its peculiarities and laws.[91] Meanwhile, Bazan has become one of the international neuropsychoanalytic tenors and has published on this subject with clock-like regularity ever since. She is one of the Ghent Freudo-Lacanians who awarded Solms an honorary doctorate and the Sarton medal even in *tempore non suspectu.*[92] Her original contributions and the position she took *vis-à-vis* Solms are discussed at the end of this book. She is considered a figurehead of Lacanian orientation, prioritising the importance of the signifier, historicity and repetition as core psychoanalytic concepts. She does talk about Freud's unconscious rather than his Id. Solms sometimes wastes no more than a single sentence on this specifically human trait: '*Humans also have a large (cortico-thalamic) capacity to satisfy their needs in imaginary and symbolic ways*'.[93] This contrasts the bulk of psychoanalytic literature, which almost exclusively treats and traverses this imaginary and symbolic space. We will see that it is encoded (coordinated by the hippocampus) mainly in the cortical tissues. Neuroscientists, then, also consider these random-access memory space.[94] It gets its charge and content at the neuronal level because of our senses and the limbic and brain stem structures responsible for our emotional arousal.[95]

Instinctive and innate behaviour is merely dispositional. It gains *incentive* only through an experience (or event-)dependent[96] dopaminergic inscription; in other words, according to history. After all, repetition is purely a result of arousal, independent of pleasure/unpleasure, value or valence because it can arise from trauma *and* pleasure. An important motive for our action in both cases is to arrive at a (this time) active performance of what had initially surprised us (both pleasantly and unpleasantly). In Bazan's neuro-Lacanian view, we will see how language and signifiers make such a big difference.

While Lacan's 'ontological dualism' conceives of language and subjectivity on the one hand and corporeality on the other as two separate orders with their logic, I (like Bazan) will not go as far as Lacan in this radicalism that I think is too divided,[97] and I will adopt an epistemological dualism. Even in this view, the body and brain can limit but not determine us. Above all, the signifiers to be historicised and contextualised cause a repetition that leads man (more than he likes) in his doings. According to some, also beyond (or even against) adaptation.[98]

Endnotes

1 Working within a clinical psychotherapy setting (psychoanalytic hospitalisation-based treatment for [posttraumatic and other] anxiety, mood and personality-disordered patients), I have been moving in this in-between zone for thirty years (Kinet 2006a). The setting I installed is inspired by my internship in the clinical psychotherapy setting as described by Verhaest, Pierloot and Janssens (1982) and Vermote and Vansina-Cobbaert (2019). Still, it is much more a-select than described there.

2 For the cover of the first Dutch-language edition of *De Geest van de Drift. Over Neuropsychoanalyse* (2022d) I designed a Rubin illusion with the vase delineated between Freud's profile. In his *The Parallax View*, Slavoj Žižek (2006) discusses the apparent displacement of an object (the shift of its position against a background) that occurs as a result of taking a different point of view. For example, he gives the wave-particle duality of quantum physics and the mind and brain dichotomy. The parallax is the gap consisting of two points between which there is no synthesis, leading to an impossible short-circuit of levels that never touch. See also Kinet (2011a).

3 It is a hobbyhorse that I have already ridden on several occasions (e.g. Kinet 2006, 2017), and I discovered only late that Bazan (2011a, 2018, Bazan and Detandt 2017) and I agree on this. Theoretically: natural as well as cultural causality, clinically: if we always hear the same sounds in violin playing, this could be due to both the instrument and the score.

4 Bazan (2014a, 2016b).

5 Solms and Turnbull (2002, pp. 56–58), Solms (2021d, pp. 301, 578).

6 Of course, this also refers to the famous distinction already made by Wilhelm Dilthey (1988 [1883]) between *erklären* and *verstehen*, explaining and understanding, characterising the natural sciences and humanities, respectively.

7 Likewise, this book navigates constantly and carefully between nature and culture.

8 Mulisch (2010).

9 Solms and Turnbull (2011).

10 Kandel (2012).

11 Kandel (1998, 1999).

12 Balchin et al. (2019).

13 In the 1940s and 1950s, psychoanalysis experienced its hay-days and was the leading model within psychiatry (Strozier 2001). With the introduction of psychopharmaceuticals and the rise of (symptom-focused) behavioural therapy (which is more in line with the medical model), it fell into decline.

14 A nice comparison from Dijksterhuis (2008). You have to make do with derivatives or traces. See also Lichtenberg (2013).

15 Lacan in his Seminar *Les formations de l'inconscient* (1998 lesson, 10/06/58).

16 To Lacan (1973, 1975a), the unconscious, drive, repetition and transference are the four fundamental concepts of psychoanalysis. In this book, the first three of them will be elaborated extensively. As for transference: at the beginning of psychoanalysis is transference. There is no intersubjectivity because between the two partners, the transference

figure (as *le sujet-supposé-savoir*/the subject-supposed-to-know) acts as a 'third' and as a pivot where everything that goes on in the transference is articulated. What speech has constructed in the past can be deconstructed in the cure by speech. It is a purely symbolic experience allowing for a reshaping of the affective and imaginary. In a first and straightforward definition, the symbolic is a semiotic system of differences and distinctions.

17 Shakespeare, *Hamlet*, Act 2, Scene 2: *Though this be madness, yet there is method in 't.*

18 Lacan (1973) on *la science du particulier* (the science of the particular) in his Seminar *Encore*, dated 8/05/1973.

19 From January 1964 onwards, Lacan gave his seminar at the Paris *Ecole Nationale Supérieure* where he talks about the censorship of his teachings and his excommunication (cf. Spinoza) from the psychoanalytic 'synagogue'. He does so before a public of intellectuals and celebrities (like Louis Althusser and Claude Lévi-Strauss) and raises many questions on the scientific status (or calling) of psychoanalysis.

20 De Gaulejac (2013).

21 Wei Zhang (2022). Two major empirical developments arising from psychoanalytic theory occurred contemporaneously: the evolution of attachment theory and the formalisation of a method for systematically observing infants in the service of diagnosis and treatment. Earlier concepts in psychoanalytic theory (e.g. Klein's paranoid–schizoid position or Bion's projective identification) provided a valuable counterpoint to reductionist views. While metaphor may have some explanatory or clarifying functions and is a handy clinical tool, it alone does not constitute science. By contrast, the work of more empirically oriented psychoanalysts (e.g. John Bowlby, Mary Ainsworth or Mary Main) or infant researchers (e.g. Beatrice Beebe, Daniel Stern, Colin Trevarthen or Edward Tronick) has provided a rich tapestry of knowledge about infant development (Kenny 2013, 2019). Some fundamental tenets, like, Winnicott's *primary maternal preoccupation* and Kohut's *mirroring*, find their incarnation in empirically validated theories of infant development, for example, Trevarthen's *primary intersubjectivity*, Stern's *cross-modal attunement* and Beebe's *micro-analyses of mother–infant communication*. Notwithstanding the strong points of convergence described, there are also significant divergences between developmental science and psychoanalytic theorising. The notion that all babies pass through auto-erotic, autistic/symbiotic, autistic-contiguous or undifferentiated, fused or merged states before emerging with a differentiated sense of self and other is still passionately embraced despite the now abundant 'evidence' to the contrary (Stern 1985, 1995). Or is this difference merely due to a confusion of tongues between a subjective and an objective stance? Every organism interacts with its environment, but this is no proof of its being a subject.

22 Westen et al. (2002, p. 88). In the psychoanalytic encounter/undertaking, the psychotherapist forms (working) hypotheses that are tested through trial interpretations and where the productive/confirming/disconfirming effect (or its absence) on subsequent free association helps to refine or correct the hypothesis. In this sense, clinical work itself has an experimental design. It is not objective but subjective 'data' that are tested/falsified/verified.

23 Grünbaum (1984). In a nutshell, I will sketch the ideal recipe for an un-scientific psychoanalysis: a hagiographic adherence to faulty theory, application of this flawed theory to therapeutic intervention, failures of the processes of observation, unencumbered by theory, restricted membership to cult-like enclaves that create closed feedback loops, whereby there is an injunction against dissent from within the group and reluctance to admit new ideas, theories or practices from without, extreme forms of conformity that tend to occur in homogeneous groups when a powerful and charismatic group leader is insistent on strict adherence to their approaches and interpretations and last but not least (cf. Popper and Grünbaums's critique) a failure to apply the scientific method, in

particular, unwillingness to subject one's theories and practices to scientific scrutiny by independent researchers, including the assessment of replicability.

24 The other major philosophy-of-science critique came from Karl Popper (2014 [1963]), who denounced the non-falsifiability of psychoanalytic assumptions. Solms, from his neuroscience angle, tries to answer both criticisms.

25 Lacan (1953a, p. 247). Psychoanalysis has only one medium: the patient's speech (a translation I prefer to the word because non-verbal utterances are also included).

26 De Kesel (2005).

27 '*Copernic et Darwin n'ont pas touché à la consistence du savoir, même s'ils en ont radicalement modifié les contenus*' (Castanet 2022, p. 11). Copernicus and Darwin didn't harm the consistency of knowledge, although they changed its contents radically (my translation). On subversion, see also Lacan (2011a, p. 22).

28 From this first Seminar (1953–1954) on the technical writings of Freud, Lacan introduces his three orders. In his second Seminar (1954–1955) and his text on Edgar Allan Poe's *The purloined letter* (1966), this Trinity replaces e the Freudian Id/Ego/Superego model. The imaginary order links the (specular) Ego with the small (mirror) other, where. In contrast, the symbolic order links the subject (S, Freud's Es) with the big Other of law and language and this link will be constitutive for the subject to be. The big Other *makes* the subject outside the subject's awareness. For the biopsychosocial (I prefer bio-socio-psychic) model, see Engel (1962).

29 The not (yet) speaking child.

30 For an extensive discussion, see Verhaeghe (2002, 2004), and Kinet (2006a, 2008b).

31 I read the oeuvre of psychoanalytic authors not so much as a (would-be) scribe. The psychoanalytic canon is not a kind of Holy Scripture. We should not adopt Luther's maxim: *Sola Scriptura*! For example, in his XI Seminar Jacques Lacan was suspicious of the rapport between psychoanalysis and religion. At the end of his teaching he dissolved his school in a letter, dated 5/1/1980, published in *Le Monde* and in it he stated: '*Il y a un problème de l'École…Ce problème se démontre tel, d'avoir une solution : c'est la dis - la dissolution … On sait ce qu'il en a coûté, que Freud ait permis que le groupe psychanalytique l'emporte sur le discours, devienne Église*'. My translation: There is a problem in the School … This problem denounces that it has a solution: the dis – the dissolution … One knows at what cost Freud has permitted the psychoanalytic community to win over discourse and thus to become a Church'. Beginning with the canon, I am constantly looking for inspirations/maps to orient myself in the clinical situation with the patient, as for the Real. As with Freud, there are different periods in Lacan's evolving oeuvre. In the first period, he talked about the Imaginary and the mirror stage, and ethological inspirations were paramount. In the second period, there was the Lacan of Symbolic order and the unconscious structured as a language. In the third period, there was the Lacan of the Real, of Thing, drive, *jouissance* and *sinthome*. This *sinthome* is an increasingly singular way of finding an 'answer' to the encounter with the Real and in the process detaching oneself both from the conventions of the big Other(s) of family and culture and from an (ideal) image of undividedness. To Lacan, the Real is by definition what cannot be symbolised. In this sense, it is the impossible, in its noumenal capacity unknowable and unnameable as a nameless being. This logical/philosophical Real drills a hole in knowing and can only be expressed, as it were, in the form of an (algebraic) unknown. In this context, the Belgian cultural philosopher Marc De Kesel speaks of 'Du Trou: X' (English: On the Hole: x) (referring to Marc Dutroux, a child rapist and murderer (of his child hostages) who held my country (Belgium) in thrall in the 1990s). To make the real a bit tangible: imagine the invisible man who can only become noticeable if paint is thrown at him or I can borrow a nice comparison from Slavoj Žižek (1991, 1997). He compares the Lacanian Real to the vanishing point in a painting. It is itself inconceivable and at the same time constitutive of any representation. He also contrasts (the beauty of) reality with

(the ugliness of) the Real. The latter is horror. It is (not the silence, but) the *crying* of the lambs. Our inner narrative is a lie and/or a defence against this Real.

32 Ockham's razor is the pursuit of the simplest possible explanatory hypothesis. Famous one-liner by this fourteenth century thinker: '*Entia non sunt multiplicanda praeter necessitatem*'. My (free) translation: If you have two competing ideas to explain the same phenomenon, you should prefer the simpler one.

33 It is the mother who introduces the infant to the symbolic or alternatively excludes him from it; Lacan calls the latter foreclosure and to him, it is the central mechanism of psychosis. He adds that it is with reference to the child's father, but a symbolised father, the dead father or the Name-of-the-Father (*le Nom-du-Père*), that the mother introduces her offspring into the order of the symbolic. For a thorough exploration of the three orders/registers, I refer to Declercq (2000) for the Real and to Van Haute (1990) for the Symbolic and the Imaginary. See also later in this book/these endnotes.

34 Nieweg (2005).

35 Jaspers (1913).

36 Schotte (2006).

37 Green (1995).

38 De Kroon (2004), Van Hoorde (2010, p. 34).

39 Lacan (1950).

40 Verhaeghe (2009).

41 Outward can also be inside the body, as it is in hypochondria or cancerophobia, for example.

42 Vandenberghe (2009).

43 Van Belzen (1988, p. 17).

44 Sacks (1984, p. 164).

45 Mooij (2002, p. 179).

46 Seminowicz et al. (2004), Etkin et al. (2005), Mayberg (2007).

47 Chalmers (1995b).

48 Solms and Turnbull (2002, p. 299).

49 It used to be the case that without psychoanalytic training, you could hardly become a clinical psychology or psychiatry professor. Nowadays the opposite is probably true.

50 Solms (2021d, p. 26).

51 Blass and Carmeli (2007).

52 Blass and Carmeli (2015). This second text is their reaction to the neuropsychoanalytic defence by Yovell, Solms and Fotopoulou (2015) against their earlier critique/accusations. Blass and Carmeli's comment is pertinent and profound, especially on dubious arguments stemming from a clinical case. They quote Freud (1926d, p. 194): 'It will soon be clear what the mental apparatus is, but I must beg you not to ask what material it is constructed of. That is not a subject of psychological interest. Psychology can be as indifferent to it as, for instance, optics can be to whether the walls of a telescope are made of metal or cardboard. We shall leave entirely on one side the material line of approach'. See note 62 for a similar statement by Lacan's stepson and editor of his Seminars Jacques-Alain Miller.

53 I mentioned elsewhere the famous 'identity pre-occupation' within the psychoanalytic world (Zenoni 1991, Kinet 2010c). What is (the pure gold of) real/authentic psychoanalysis?

54 Verhaeghe (1991) elaborates Jacques Lacan's discourse theory in detail. Simply put, there is the master discourse (the speaker speaks from his knowledge), the university discourse (the speaker speaks from institutionalised knowledge), the hysterical discourse (the speaker speaks from his suffering/lack) and the analytic discourse (the speaker suspends his knowledge in a learned ignorance). These discourses rotate among themselves, but only the last discourse is typical of psychoanalytic therapy forms and keeps the psychoanalytic process's engine running.

55 Shevrin (2010).
56 Verhaeghe (2012, p. 224).
57 Freud (1895a, p. 295; 1895b, p. 225).
58 See most recently Castanet (2022, p. 12). The microscope is a precious scientific tool, but not to look at the sky. For this, the giant ear of the satellite dish is better suited.
59 For example Jos Dirkx, Jos de Kroon, Michel Thys or Paul Verhaeghe.
60 For example Antonie Ladan, Nelleke Nicolai, Marc Hebbrecht or Rudi Vermote.
61 The *International Psychoanalytical Association* is mainly Anglo-Saxon (Ego-psychology, object relations theory, (post-) Kleinians, Bionians but also Lacanians) while the *Association Mondiale de Psychanalyse* is almost exclusively Lacanian. There is a sharp divide between the two despite the (attempted) dialogue initiated by their respective presidents Horacio Etchegoyen and Lacan's son-in-law, Jacques-Alain Miller (1996). In their diatribe, Miller bristles at the relevance of neurocorrelations. To him, it matters as much (or as little) that the mind would know a correlate in the mind of God.
62 I often refer to them simply as the Anglos and Latins.
63 Kinet (2010b).
64 Luyten (2019, p. 6).
65 Verhaeghe (2010).
66 Gould (1981).
67 McCabe and Castel (2008), Weisberg et al. (2008).
68 After the title of Verhaeghe's chapter in our book (2010) *Geestdrift voor het Brein* (Geest=mind, drift = drive, brein=brain).
69 Lacan (1953a, p. 259).
70 Fink (1997).
71 Porge (1989).
72 See, e.g., Green (1995), Mooij (2002), Schotte (2006), and Van Hoorde (2010).
73 Feys (2009, p. 63).
74 Dirkx (2016).
75 Swaab (2010).
76 Changeux (1983).
77 Nietzsche (2004 [1886]).
78 Kinet (2019).
79 Haraway (2015). For millennia, humanity barely caused nature any harm. Only with the industrial revolution and capitalism have we begun to deplete/destroy each other and Mother Earth.
80 Kapuszinsky (2006), from whom I summarise and paraphrase a passage.
81 Groddeck (1977).
82 The small other and especially the big Other will come back even more often. From his second seminar onward (1988b, pp. 275–288), Lacan distinguishes between this small other and big Other, and the psychoanalyst, in his view, must always keep this distinction strictly in mind. The small other or a is the other as similar. He is both alter-ego and mirror image and belongs fully to the imaginary (quasi-ethological) register of mirror(-ing), attachment and seduction. The big Other or A is the Other in its radical alterity and is equated by Lacan with the law or language and belongs to the symbolic order. He emphasises that this language comes from elsewhere. Indeed, it is the mother tongue originating from that (usually) first big Other, the *(M)Other.* In a paraphrase of Descartes: *Elle pense, donc je suis.* 'She thinks, therefore I am' or in a famous Lacanian slogan: the unconscious is the discourse of the Other. In its broader sense, the big Other is the treasury of the signifier and the culture that determines how we eat, sleep, dress, enjoy, die and so on. The advantage of these abstract and invariant terms is that they permanently lend themselves to culturally variant interpretations.
83 Lacan (1986, pp. 64, 75).
84 Verhaeghe (2010).

85 *Je fais partie de ceux qui ne font pas de partie* (I am part of those who don't form a party, my translation), but although I am not (and certainly not a full-blooded) Lacanian, the word signifier will come up often. The distinction between signifier and signified is essential within Lacanian psychoanalysis. It comes in a modified sense from the work of the linguist Ferdinand de Saussure (2002 [1916]). Indeed, the signifier does not appear in Freud's work as a concept. As an initially meaningless and purely material/phonetic element, it is given primacy (logically rather than chronologically) by Lacan. Signifiers are basic elements of language that differ among themselves. They do not express pre-existing meaning but produce meaning according to context (in the clinical situation: the diachronic context of narration and the synchronic context of the transference–countertransference). To Lacan, language is not a system of signs but of signifiers. The field of these signifiers is the field of the big Other. According to Lacan, the unconscious does not precede or underlie ('pre-verbal') language, but conversely is instead its result or effect. In this sense, only man as a speaking being has an unconscious. The Lacanian psychoanalyst will first and foremost listen to what the analysand (does not) say rather than to what he (allegedly) would *like to* say.

86 Verhaeghe (2015).

87 Ter Balkt (2000). Dutch and English version https://www.poetryinternational.com/nl/poets-poems/poem/103-13805_THE-ANIMAL-CRUSADE#lang-en

88 Van Coillie (2022).

89 According to Noam Chomsky, humans are evolutionarily pre-wired for language. This 'organ' explains a kind of *universal grammar*. See, for example, Cook and Newson (2014).

90 Stortelder and Goetmakers-Burg (2010).

91 Kinet (2010c).

92 Solms received the Sarton medal in 1996. See Balchin et al. (2019, p. 92) in which many international neuropsychoanalysts testify to twenty years of neuropsychoanalytic evolutions.

93 Solms (2018b, p. 6).

94 Solms (2021f, pp. 560–56).

95 For details, see Ellis and Solms (2018).

96 Bazan often uses the word 'event' which refers to Alain Badiou with his *L'Etre et L'Evénément* (1988) and where he (inspired by Lacan) considers the act or event as an inaugural or constitutive moment for subjectification.

97 Kinet (2010b).

98 Famous example: Van Haute (2000), whose *Against Adaptation* not only explains Lacan's famous *graphe du désir* step by step but also criticises extensively all too naive notions of adaptation. In short: adaptation is a biological concept whereby organisms are supposed to be driven to adapt themselves to fit the environment. As such a harmony between the inner and the surrounding world is presupposed. Ego-psychology, in particular, explains neurotic symptoms in terms of maladaptive behaviour and psychoanalytic treatment should help patients to better adapt to reality. Lacan opposes every attempt to explain human phenomena solely in terms of adaptation (Lacan 1966, pp. 158, 171–172). Reality is not a simple, objective given to which the Ego must adapt, but it is precisely a product of the Ego's fictional misrepresentations. There is an illusory sense of adaptation that blocks access to the unconscious. Secondly, the analyst is not the arbiter of the patient's adaptation (nor his own) nor does he in any way impose his power. Finally – and because of his inscription in the symbolic order – man is a part of but also apart from nature. There is a 'gap' (Lacan 1988b, p. 323). See later in this book.

Chapter 4

Interlude

Psychoanalytic Wit

Freud wrote (in addition to his job behind the couch) some eight thousand pages, and Winston Churchill wrote more than Walter Scott and Charles Dickens combined. Freud was awarded the Goethe Prize and Churchill the Nobel Prize for Literature. You could easily compile an anthology of witty one-liners from both gentlemen. They will get laughs, and what psychoanalyst does not use a *captatio benevolentiae* from time to time to warm up his unruly audience?

Not much has changed since Freud. In his letter to Wilhelm Fliess of November 5, 1897, he writes: 'My classes are attended by eleven students who sit there with pen and paper and who, unfortunately, hear little positive from me'.[1] Or in his May 2, 1935 letter to Arnold Zweig: 'The times are dark. Fortunately, it is not my job to brighten them'.[2] Freud also constantly makes brilliant use of metaphors. An entire section in *Sigmund Freud Werken* is devoted to them.[3] Their reading is a pithy alternative to many introductions to psychoanalysis.

Take this rambling selection of loose chatter. On several occasions, Freud compares the psychoanalyst to a surgeon who must wield the scalpel with cold-bloodedness to separate the healthy from the diseased tissue. He compares them to the radiologist who is exposed to dangerous radiation and must sometimes bear the harmful consequences of it. He compares them to an archaeologist who tries to reconstruct prehistory based on stones and bones. He compares them to a mirror that – opaque – only reflects on what is offered.

What's more: there is the psychoanalyst who, like Sancho Panza, confronts Don Quixote with his romantic delusions of meaning.[4] Or the psychoanalyst who resembles a court jester: his half-witted remarks is the only mouth from which His Majesty (the Ego) accepts less pleasant truths. I refer to this connection to the widely known cynical joke. The neurotic builds castles in the air, the psychotic inhabits them and the psychiatrist rakes in the money.

More still: in connection with the timing of the interpretation, I especially like this one: the lion only jumps once. This is related to the patient's resistance, making him a monarch who takes advice from his courtiers instead of listening to the people. Or like a child who does not want to open his clenched fist to show what is inside because it is undoubtedly something wrong, something he should not have. A last one: our consciousness behaves like a man who rushes to the attic after a

DOI: 10.4324/9781003394358-4

suspicious noise in the basement only to find that he had imagined something. In contrast, the brave man does not dare venture into the dark.

Jacques Lacan compares the psychoanalyst to the dead man (*'le mort'*) in the game of bridge, who always keeps his cards covered. Slavoj Žižek compares him to a detective. There are nota bene, two types of detective. Sherlock Holmes, who works with cerebral detachment, and Philip Marlowe, who – whether or not urged to do so by some *femme fatale* – ventures into some heart of darkness, risking life and limb. Admittedly, both move between art and science. Paraphrasing the French poet René Char *'le scientifique cherche des preuves et l'artiste des traces'*.[5] The scientist seeks proof, and the artist traces. And how about this one-liner: psychoanalysis is the science of traces?

Following a postmodern adage, why not combine high and low culture? I sometimes compare the psychoanalyst to a miner. He works deep underground and in darkness. He has good night vision because he is more accustomed than any other to what never sees the light of day. Or comparing psychoanalysis to specific household tasks. Instead of talking about being in O (Wilfred Bion)[6] or identifying with object little a as the cause of desire (Jacques Lacan),[7] why not compare ourselves to a vacuum cleaner?

In his 1647 *Manual, Oracle*, Baltasar Gracian says, 'Prescribing something or nothing requires the same amount of learning from a physician'.[8] It would be best if you had as much wit to do/say nothing as to do/say something. You are just cleverly keeping yourself dumb. Silence is an action or punctuation like any other. The best way to get someone to speak is to be silent. That way, the material gets sucked up. From under the carpet, too.

Instead of interpretation, I suggest the can opener. Through the cracks or crevices in (the tin cans of) speaking, it provides insight into contents that are as yet sealed off. Even when their storage date has passed, toxic gases begin or threaten to escape. With this simple tool, we can open or expand the gaze. Thus, we can notice repetitive things against which the memory of their roots can provide excellent antidotes. Finally, we use the metaphor of ironing. All wrinkles and folds (false or otherwise) have formed in us over time. One thing is examining the folds and where, when and from whom they come. To iron them out of our system, we must go over them repeatedly – as every ironer knows in various ways and from multiple angles.

Psychotherapy is using thought to come to a better understanding of and grip on feelings. More updated ones can replace old automatisms with varying degrees of success.

Should the reader wonder why I started with Winston Churchill, it is simply because of a famous excerpt from his 1947 speech in the House of Commons. I quote, 'No one pretends that democracy is perfect or all-wise. Indeed, it has been said that democracy is the worst form of government except for all those other forms that have been tried from time to time'.[9] One could replace 'democracy' with 'psychoanalysis' and 'government' with 'treatment', and you would get the point.

Endnotes

1 Masson (1985, p. 277).
2 Letter to Zweig (Freud 1961, p. 425).
3 Freud (2006, pp. 454–473). All of these famous Freudian metaphors come from this Index.
4 Phillips (2014, p. 42).
5 Char (1983, p. 382).
6 O of Bion: the zone of unknowable and unattainable ultimate truth. See, recently, Vermote (2018) and more particularly, Alisobhani and Corstorphine (2019).
7 The object a is the object-cause of desire. It is (the image of) a lost object that is repeatedly sought but never found. It is small a of the small (and not the big) other: the other-similar as projection or reflection of the ego or (perhaps better) of the self. The term is left untranslated. Like x or n(x), it is an algebraic unknown that plays an important role in all kinds of Lacanian 'mathemes'.
8 Gracian (2016 [1647] aphorism 138).
9 Churchill (2001, p. 19).

Chapter 5

Neuropsychoanalysis

Neuropsychoanalysis

Could neuropsychoanalysis create an overarching framework, integrating insights from neuroscience with a psychoanalytic focus on subjective experience? Could it lead to a kind of 'Theory of Everything/TOE' that, for example, physics is also striving for? Big question mark, given that it is prey to an inner gap or division. It can contribute to more integration between the various psychoanalytic perspectives (e.g. of drive, Ego, object, self, mentalisation, attachment and so on) that are equally trying to design maps for the field of the psyche. Many psychoanalytic authors[1] resist an excessive postmodern pluralism in which various Great (metapsychological) Narratives can coexist. Philosophy, politics, ethics or art may revolve around the same questions over and over again. Which, by the way, makes them both frustrating and fascinating for many. The answer changes constantly, and progress is far from guaranteed. Science and technology, on the other hand, are cumulative. Knowledge accumulates. That heliocentrism and geocentrism cannot go together is evident in the (natural) sciences. Technology, too, does not reverse. We no longer ride in a horse-drawn cart. The Internet has replaced the carrier pigeon. Bloodlettings are things of the past. Psychoanalysis holds a peculiar position in this, too. For instance, its clinical insights are often timeless. Even clinicians of the first hour (besides Freud Karl Abraham, for example, or Sandor Ferenczi)[2] still have much to teach a contemporary psychoanalyst. At the same time, the advances of psychoanalysis as a science are primarily cumulative.

Neuropsychoanalysis, in any case, tries to remedy the overly simplistic reductions of neuroscience. Every philosophy of mind[3] espouses such anti-reductionist views. Yet, it is still being debated whether neuroscientific tenors avoid this trap altogether.[4] Where in the brain would the subject (as a thinking thing/*res cogitans*) be located? Descartes' anachronistic hypothesis that it would be found in the pineal gland should not be replaced by substantially similar (albeit much more complex) reductions because 'There's nobody there!' Thoughts, feelings and desires are products of persons, not brains.[5] In this context, Solms often quotes Oliver Sacks: 'It is precisely the subject, the living "I", which is excluded from neurology'.[6]

Dixit philosopher Francis Bacon 'Nature is conquered only by obedience'.[7] Neuropsychoanalysis could counter naive views on the interaction between genes

DOI: 10.4324/9781003394358-5

and the environment.[8] It could then make it clear that the environment should be understood not as the actual but as the subjective environment.[9] How the environment is perceived and what we have made of it acts as a filter in the expression of genotype into phenotype, i.e. in the translation of genetic potential into personality and behaviour.[10] On the other hand, neuropsychoanalysis seeks to avoid the shadowy mythology and speculative shortcomings of psychoanalytic metapsychology by grounding its theorising more in empirical data. For instance, distilling drive theory from listening to the free association on the sofa led Freud to miraculous insights. But isn't there much to learn about the life of the drive from entirely different observations from outside the consulting room, too?

Neuropsychoanalysts advocate cooperation between psychoanalysis and neuroscience and not incorporation. Physiology and psychology should be studied separately, and correlations can be sought afterwards. There should be mutual respect for respective methodological and epistemological limitations.[11] The material monism employed by neuroscience often remains somewhat reductionist: 'Mind is what brain does'. Dutch-language neuroscientist Dick Swaab perhaps takes the biscuit in this reductionism. For him, the mind is an excretion product: the brain's urine.[12] In contrast, neuropsychoanalysts harbour a modified monism called 'dual aspect monism'[13] or supervenience physicalism.[14] The mind originates in the brain, which, after all, acts as a material condition. The brain can be objectively and scientifically examined from the outside, but the free association is a competent research tool where we can observe our experience from within.[15]

Neuroscience has abundantly proven that most mental processes belong in the (descriptive) category of the non-conscious.[16] This non-conscious should be distinguished from the Freudian unconscious in a narrower sense.[17] The latter is classically the repressed or psychodynamic and pulsational systemic unconscious that functions according to the (fluid) mode of the primary process. It knows neither time nor contradiction, pleasure principle and psychic reality prevail, and processes of condensation and displacement replace logic *and* rationale.[18] Mark Solms sometimes succinctly calls the primary process a fancy way of saying that you still ignore logic and contradiction and don't distinguish past from present or thoughts from actions. It is, according to him, consciousness without the rules of reality applied.

Neuroplasticity

Lifelong neuroplasticity is undoubtedly the most crucial neuroscientific discovery. It contradicts any static or fatalistic view of the brain.[19] 'Your brain makes your being, but your being also makes your brain'.[20] This neuroplasticity is the result of synaptogenesis, especially in the first three years of life and (at the level of the cortex) in puberty, dendrites growing and branching out, axons lengthening and branching out, pruning, myelination of axons, faster synapses, decrease in inhibition, neurogenesis, etc. Learning creates functional networks that are rapidly stimulated by certain things. Cells that fire together wire together. The so-called Hebbian plasticity plays a role in learning, making specific neuronal processes faster and more efficient.[21]

There is experience-independent plasticity. This involves spontaneously and internally generated processes that occur without external influence. For example,[22] I give the development of different layers in a structure at the lateral geniculate nucleus of the thalamus.[23] There is experience-dependent plasticity, depending on the life led by this or that unique person. Indeed, all experiences influence the design of neuronal conjunctions. For example, playing the violin, mental arithmetic and gymnastics leave their distinct mark on the brain.[24] Finally, there is experience-expected plasticity through a combination of genes and influence from the outside world in a standard, developmentally appropriate way that gives rise to common traits. For example, experience-expected plasticity leads to skills such as walking, command of the mother tongue, distinguishing faces and perceiving diagonals.[25]

Peter Fonagy[26] suggests that gene expression is partly dependent on the environment. He describes the 'gene–environment interaction', which defines the environment as the attachment relationship. According to Fonagy, we are endowed with a natural and evolutionary ability to develop an interpersonal, interpretive capacity: the capacity of mind-reading and understanding the mental state of the other.[27] Children only become aware of their inner state through others.[28] In a variation on Descartes: Elle *pense, donc je suis*. She (the mother) thinks, therefore, I am.[29]

Also, fMRI before and after psychotherapy shows changes at the level of the brain, as has become apparent in several studies.[30] According to Helen Mayberg, psychotherapy works top-down, with changes mainly occurring at the level of the cognitive regions. Pharmacotherapy works bottom-up with changes primarily at the limbic system and brain stem level. Symptom reduction also has a well-defined sequence[31] with psychotherapy affecting worrying and pharmacotherapy acting more on neuro-vegetative symptoms. Nothing mammalian is foreign to humans, as we read in *Nature* that all mammals share common attachment mechanisms and stress-regulating neurophysiology. Under normal conditions, early mother–child interactions facilitate the development of self-regulatory structures in the cortico-limbic region of the right hemisphere. As a result of trauma, right hemisphere dysfunction can develop. This leads to vulnerability to post-traumatic stress disorder and a greater predisposition to violence in adulthood.[32]

Attachment

Much research has been carried out on the neurobiology of attachment.[33] It is well established that the latter's quality greatly influences neuroplasticity, the calibration of corticotropin-releasing factors, and the immune system.[34] Stress in early development causes damage to sensorimotor and cognitive–emotional development.[35] Growth of the hippocampus, for example, lags due to stress.[36] Stress produces dysregulation of the hypothalamic–pituitary–adrenal (HHB) axis with impaired memory storage and reduced adaptive capacity.[37]

In cases of neglect, abuse and disorganised attachment, the development of the brain's right hemisphere and the *amygdala*, but especially the *hippocampus,* are impaired.[38] Reduced attention or prolonged separation from the mother have the same consequences.[39] Insecure attachment, on the other hand, produces increased stress sensitivity[40] and is a significant risk factor for developing borderline personality disorder.[41] Loving care is necessary for development.[42] Secure attachment increases stress resilience and sets the benchmark for our immune system.[43]

The work of Allan Schore is of exceptional importance for understanding the neurobiology of attachment and early childhood development. It combines psycho-analytic theory and mother–child observation with the use of fMRI. It turns out that the early social environment of primary caretakers directly influences brain structures, which are responsible for socio-emotional development. The developing brain depends on the nature of early childhood experiences with the caretaker, significantly affecting emotional growth. Current imaging techniques make it possible to map the development of the right hemisphere (especially the right pre-orbital frontal cortex)[44] and its role in early emotional communication and development. Visual exchange or mirror responses are of great importance here. In development, the right hemisphere is ahead until 18–36 months. Then the left hemisphere becomes dominant. When a mother interacts with *her* child, she experiences suitable hemispheric activity with *another* child's left hemispheric activity. At the time of language development, there is a spectacular increase in interhemispheric connections at the level of the *corpus callosum.*[45] Unconscious and conscious, primary and secondary processes correlate convincingly with the right and left hemispheres, respectively. Early affective experiences significantly impact the development of structures that govern unconscious information processes.[46] Freud's view that direct communication is possible between two unconsciouses is compatible with hundreds of research articles compiled by Schore.[47] They support intersubjective[48] and two-person psychology-based psychotherapeutic developments.[49]

Both Freud[50] and Lacan[51] have explicitly drawn attention to the helplessness and physiological immaturity of the human child. In Winnicott's terms, the child's first period of life is characterised by 'absolute dependence'.[52] Without the 'primary maternal pre-occupation'[53] of the matrixial mother, the infant cannot develop optimally psychologically. In this first period of life, a representational system consists of an image of self and others, crystallised around the 'arousal' or stimulation experienced by the child. Depending on the theory, this involves an 'inner working model',[54] a cognitive schema,[55] a 'self-other-affect triad',[56] proto-narrative envelopes/schemes of togetherness,[57] a particular attachment pattern,[58] and so on that define our way of being in the world. They are all fixed in procedural memory and continue to leave a decisive mark on anything and everything.[59] They then stand as a sols key for the stave, and tuning into them is of indispensable (empathic) importance for striking the right (affective) tone in the session. It is an integral part of any psychoanalytic process to bring these implicit patterns to the conscious attention of the analysand in an emotionally meaningful way. Peter Fonagy[60] even promotes this as the essential component of therapeutic practice.

Memory and Remembrance

Neuroscientific findings related to memory and recall have great relevance to psychoanalysis. After all, Freud and his contemporaries did not yet suspect the existence of various memory systems that have been mapped today. Melanie Klein, however, introduced 'memories in feeling' as indicators of implicit/procedural memory (not yet known as such in her time).[61] Some of our feelings *are* memories. Based on these feelings, we enter – as if via a time machine – directly into our (early) childhood past. Christopher Bollas spoke of the 'unthought known',[62] which can thus be (re-)constructed by the analyst during the session. Meanwhile, Schore[63] has substantiated this and similar clinical intuitions, e.g. of Bion, Winnicott, Kohut, etc.[64] All this plays a fundamental role in the mirroring elements of the therapeutic relationship and the so-called a-specific or generic therapeutic factors.[65]

I have since fully integrated the difference between implicit and explicit memory into my clinical work and theoretical views.[66] The discovery of implicit memory has dramatically expanded the concept of the unconscious.[67] It is the circuit within which emotional and affective pre-symbolic and pre-verbal experiences from the early mother–child relationship are stockpiled. They then appear to come 'live on stage' within the transference–countertransference continuum and can be analysed there. Thus, the fact that the *amygdala* matures more quickly than the *hippocampus* implies that psychoanalysts now have a more nuanced view of the unconscious and early childhood amnesia.[68] Freud's repressed unconscious (dynamic, based on repression, dependent on the hippocampus) can thus be distinguished from the non-repressed unconscious. The neural substrate of the latter unconscious would be situated at the level of the posterior associative areas of the right cerebral hemisphere and depend on connections with the *amygdala*, among others. As early as the end of pregnancy, relational and affective patterns are recorded in implicit memory. This domain of implicit memory is unconscious, not repressed and not recallable through words. The earliest experiences stored there form a structural part of this unconscious and assert their influence on adult life. In this way, they permanently influence later relationships' depth and emotional colour. They become noticeable in dreams and also through the musical dimension of speech.[69]

Memory research further distinguishes between non-conscious, a-noetic and implicit memory and explicit, biographical and declarative memory, which differ functionally and anatomically.[70] To recall memories of past events, they must first be stored in vivid memory. This explicit or declarative memory contains semantic memory on the one hand and episodic memory on the other.[71] Semantic memory involves memories encoded from the third-person perspective (e.g. the meaning of words, concepts, traffic signals and so on). Episodic or auto-noetic memory is the 'mental time travel' in which we are present as experiencing subjects either as participants or observers, for example in the case of arguments or a crush. These memories are encoded from the first-person point of view. They are both defined by their ideational character, take the form of thoughts and are encoded in cortical tissue. The *hippocampus* (cortical but more ancient than the neocortex) is of prime importance for both forms of explicit memory. This autobiographical memory also appeals to many other parts of the brain, e.g. the prefrontal cortex, anterior cingulate cortex, temporal cortex, parietal cortex and *cerebellum*.[72] Because the *hippocampus* does not mature sufficiently until three to four years after birth, a child cannot store verbally structured memories before then.[73] Many experiences have already set the tone, but we cannot narrate or retell them.

The frontal cortex retrieves memories in a realistic, rational and orderly manner and plays a crucial controlling role in imprinting and storage.[74] Before the second year of life, the frontal cortex is poorly developed, but when a child is about two years old, a substantial growth spurt occurs, followed by a second spurt around the fifth year.[75] All this makes it plausible that young children's memories are stored differently from those of adults and will also be more difficult to access later in life using the frontal system, which has altered so much since.[76]

Implicit memory is the unrepressed and unrememberable unconscious that appears only during (inter-)action and repetition.[77] It is also called procedural or 'skill and habit' memory[78] that operates, for example, in the grammatical application of the mother tongue or in walking, cycling, speaking and driving. Explicit memory, by the way, can be transformed into implicit memory through repetition.[79] The 'natural' ways a person is present in the world and interacts with others belong to the domain of implicit memory. These ways of being in the world can be understood as memories, but memories that are 'expressed' in how a person is and behaves.[80] So, this implicit knowledge is not remembered but enacted or acted out.[81] It is unconscious knowledge, not dynamically unconscious through repression, but not conscious, i.e. flowing 'naturally' beyond consciousness.[82]

Implicit memory also contains the more emotional form of memory governed by the *amygdala* and the associated areas.[83] They undergo much faster maturation than the structures involved in explicit memory.[84] The almond nucleus is connected to the *hippocampus* via two pathways and influences explicit memory. According to Joseph LeDoux, implicit memory is indelible, while on the other hand, the *hippocampus* can be damaged both as a result of trauma and separation from the mother. Conscious attention is needed to influence implicit memory (e.g. in psychotherapy). Looking ahead to the clinic, procedural and emotional memory are most relevant.[85] They have different operating principles. They are both hard to forget, but the former is hard to learn and the latter easy to learn. Indeed, for instance, on fear-inducing or sexual experiences, learning can occur even after a single exposure, and it is hard to undo.[86] Both emotional and procedural memory goes beyond thinking; according to Solms, they are characteristic of the systemic unconscious, and they thus shed a different light on Freud's repetition compulsion.[87] Such non-declarative memory traces can be reconsolidated; however, not through thinking (as conscious cognition or working memory) but only by experience. They only become labile and amenable to revision/reconsolidation through 'embodied enactment',[88] namely in the living and lived reality of the psychoanalytic encounter.

Endnotes

1 Shevrin (1995).
2 Karl Abraham who introduced the idea/concept of the bad (narcissistic) mother and the sadism that is a part of the oral and anal phase (Kinet 2015d) and Sandor Ferenczi, who pioneered the constructive use of the countertransference, who was a precursor of relational psychoanalysis and whose views of the psychodynamics and phenomenology of childhood trauma remain inspiring to this day (Kinet 2023).
3 Crane and Patterson (2001).
4 Glas (2006).
5 Den Boer (2003).
6 Sacks (1984 p 164).
7 Bacon (2000 [1620]).
8 So-called epigenetics. See, e.g., Van Reekum and Schmeets (2008).
10 Ladan (2006).
11 Fonagy (2003a, p. 236).
12 Not that this thought is new. Neuroscientist Jean-Pierre Changeux refers to philosopher and physician Cabanis in 1802: *le cerveau secrète la pensée comme le foie la bile* (1983, p. 25). The brain excretes thoughts like the liver excretes bile (my translation).
13 Mancia (2006). A monism already honoured by Spinoza in his double aspect: *natura naturans* and *natura naturata* see Damasio (2010). Another figurehead of (mind–body) monism is Bishop George Berkeley. His subjective idealism famously held that '*esse est percipi*'/to be is to be perceived. After all, there can't be a mind–body problem if there are only minds. According to Berkeley, there is only the mind and the ideas the world is made of. See https://www.earlymoderntexts.com/assets/pdfs/berkeley1710_2.pdf
14 Vandenberghe (2009).
15 Solms and Turnbull (2002, pp. 56–58); Joris Vandenberghe, Van Oudenhove, and Cuypers (2010).
16 Baars (2003a, 2003b). The descriptive unconscious largely corresponds to what Freud called the systemic pre-conscious. It is easily summoned; indeed, we do not encounter the resistance that characterises the exploration of the systemic unconscious, which is not descriptive but pulsational and dynamic.
17 Dunn (2003).
18 Freud (1900a, 1900b).
19 Doidge (2007).
20 Sitskoorn (2006, 2010).
21 Hebb (1949) in Sitskoorn (2006, p. 40).
22 The lateral geniculate nucleus is the main centre for processing visual information from the retina.
23 Sitskoorn (2006, p. 67).
24 Ibid., p. 68.
25 Ibid., p. 146.
26 Fonagy (2003b).
27 In contemporary views, this is mainly associated with mirroring, mentalisation, etc. However, this is already contained in Freud's primary experience of satisfaction. Because it is the mother who nursed the child, the child's cry becomes an adequate act *nachträglich* (due to 'afterwardsness'). The mother's interpretation/response was an essential link.
28 Fonagy and Target (1998, pp. 14–15).
29 Cluckers and Meurs (2005).
30 Seminowicz et al. (2004); Roffman et al. (2005); Mayberg (2007, pp. 729–730).
31 Goldapple et al. (2004).

32 Bradshaw et al. (2005); LaBar and Cabeza (2006).
33 Fuchs (2004).
34 Mancia (2006, p. 8).
35 Bremner (1999), Den Boer and Glas (2005, p. 19).
36 Ibid., p. 24.
37 Nicolai (2009, p. 569).
38 Ibid., p. 571.
39 Meaney (2001), De Kloet (2009, p. 547).
40 Perry (2001).
41 Herman et al. (1989).
42 den Boer and Glas (2005, p. 26).
43 Liu et al. (1997).
44 Schore (1994, 2003a, 2003b).
45 This is a prefrontal cortical region involved in the cognitive decision-making process. Because of its connection with emotions and reward, it is sometimes considered a part of the limbic system.
46 Schore (2003b, p. 244).
47 Schore (1994, p. 280).
48 Schore (2003b).
49 Whereby an analytic third (Ogden 2004) or psychoanalytic field (Ferro & Civitarese 2015) is formed within the psychoanalytic encounter as a joint co-creation of both 'players'.
50 Freud (1923a, 1923b).
51 Lacan (1949).
52 Winnicott (1960, p. 46).
53 Winnicott (1956).
54 Bowlby (1988).
55 Bucci (1997).
56 Kernberg (1976).
57 Stern (1995).
58 Main and Goldwyn (1995, pp. 237–239).
59 Kandel (1999).
60 Fonagy (1999, p. 219).
61 Klein (1957, p. 180).
62 Bollas (1987).
63 Schore (2003a, 2003b).
64 Kinet (2008b, 2009b).
65 Kinet (2009a, 2010c).
66 Kinet (2006a, 2008b, 2009b, 2010c).
67 Mancia (2006).
68 Eichenbaum (1998, 1999, pp. 775–776).
69 Ogden (1999), Mancia (2006, p. 9). To Adam Phillips, psychoanalysis is not a science, nor should it aspire to be one. To him, it's a kind of 'practical poetry' (1994, p. xi). I think he confuses psychoanalysis as a therapeutic practice with the evolving knowledge of the specific laws of the unconscious/the subject/the human psyche.
70 Schacter (1996, 2001).
71 Andreasen et al. (1995).
72 Where everything called the 'cortex' is the more evolved and the cerebellum a subcortical, evolutionarily older structure (on top of the 'brain stem') that serves mainly motor coordination and balance.
73 Sitskoorn (2006).

74 Ladan (2000).
75 Solms and Turnbull (2002)
76 Ladan (2006).
77 Solms and Turnbull (2002).
78 Ladan (2000, p. 26).
79 Mancia (2006, p. 41).
80 Kandel (2006) Well-known example is driving a car at first explicitely and then automated/implicitely.
81 Ladan (2006).
82 Clyman (1991).
83 Fonagy (1999), Mancia (2006), Ladan (2006).
84 Ibid., p. 252.
85 Ibid., p. 242.
86 Solms (2018c).
87 Ibid.
88 Ibid.

Chapter 6

Interlude

Pygmalion

Bernard is the middle of three brothers. Father has a militaristic disposition and insists on discipline. Bernard barely felt seen by his mother's eyes. She once bluntly crushed his boyhood dream of becoming a fighter pilot. This memory is prototypical. It is a model for countless examples of hurtful mirroring he received from her. From childhood, he has been an *Einzelgänger*. During his psychotherapy, the image of a (Un-)Lucky Luke[1] emerged: a poor, lonesome cowboy a long way from home.

Bernard makes many distant journeys but is paradoxically in search of a motherland, a place where he can come home. Socially, it has always been one against all in his emotional world. He lives entirely according to his rigid principles, averse to his entourage. Now in his forties, he is still single and lives again with his parents. He barely leaves his room and only has computer contact with the outside world. He has been coming to the clinic weekly for years, but since the COVID-19 pandemic, our sessions are digital at his request.

An incident from when he was on a school trip to the Alps has come up several times. His classmates were chatting and laughing on a terrace. He turned away from the group to enjoy the cold mountain air and snowy peaks. His way of speaking is always very abstract and rational. One of the higher studies he tried was mathematics. He loves its purity. He also plays with the literal meaning. The art of cutting.[2] He then realises that this has to do with erasing negative reflections that befell him from his mother.

In his elementary school days, a girl lived across the street. She often sat on the second floor behind the window and smiled every time she saw him. That gave him a warm feeling. In the course of therapy, it turns out that the image of this young lady (whom he at one point called his Mona Lisa) set the tone, so to speak, for his relating to women. Thus, to this day, he is an avid photographer. He makes prints of impressions. In doing so, he is primarily on the lookout for female models. Not for glamour, nor for erotic pictures, but he has a female (ideal) image in mind that he tries to realise with the cooperation of these ladies. He makes close-ups of ladies playing sports. Paraphrasing German philosopher Friedrich Schiller:[3] is man (in this case: a woman) ever more authentic than when he (she) is at play?

DOI: 10.4324/9781003394358-6

For his photo shoots, he spares neither expense nor effort. However, he does nothing with the photos. At least nothing public or economic. They only play a role in his inner world. He draws on them. I was more reminded of icons: the famous panels from the Greek Orthodox Church depicting the Madonna and Child. During our sessions, the title of the feature film *Et Dieu créa la femme* also often came to my mind. Or I thought of the Pygmalion theme elaborated by the Irish playwright George Bernard Shaw, which became known to the broader public through the blockbuster musical *My Fair Lady*. The artist or professor falls in love with the image he has created.

Pygmalion is a Cypriot prince portrayed by Ovid in his Metamorphoses (X, 243–267). Disappointed by his experience with bad women, he remains a bachelor and creates an ivory statue of a (dream of a) woman: Galatea. She is at once a mother-virgin and a spirit-daughter who awakens like a Sleeping Beauty under his sculpting fingers. Like *Her* (in the feature film of the same name), she is the consummate product of male imagination.

In doing so, the man places or sees a mysterious 'something', a *je-ne-sais-quoi* in his beloved. It is, according to Jacques Lacan, pure sublimation. In his winged formulation: the art – or love – object is elevated to the dignity of the (maternal and incestuous) Thing. The words and images with which he clothes her serve at once to maintain the gap with this Thing as to bridge it. The beloved or the work of art is a dream image: wishful thinking or mirage in which the object (small a) that causes desire seems hidden. I translate this to the musical. In reality, Eliza Doolittle (who matters little) is elevated by the linguistics professor Henry Higgins to a beloved Duchess with whom he can show off in High Society.

In the more recent feature film *Her*, the Intuitive Operating System (portrayed under the name Samantha by Scarlett Johansson) knows enough after just one communication. When romantic-letter writer and main character Theodore Twombly (Joaquin Phoenix) wants to tell his mother something, he complains that she always starts talking about herself. This frustrates him. It is enough information for Samantha to seamlessly tune in, fully responding to all that Theodore says, does or desires. A passionate infatuation is the logical consequence of this perfect mirroring. It is a fine example of what Slavoj Žižek alludes to virtual reality is well suited to alert us to the virtual aspect of any 'reality', including that of love.

That Shaw elaborated on the Pygmalion theme may be associated with the early loss of (the love of) his mother.[4] The narcissistic factor in the Pygmalion phenomenon is also evident.[5] Returning to the clinic, Bernard had a great passion in his young adulthood: Ella.[6] He was crazy about her and completely lost himself in a passionate infatuation. Until she rejected him, and he fell into a severe depression that necessitated psychiatric hospitalisation. More or less consciously, afterwards, he defensively turned away from any amorous opening. This is under the motto: not twice. Many a psychoanalyst would correct this (perhaps tacitly): not thrice…

Endnotes

1 *Lucky Luke* is a Western *bande dessinée* (comic book) series created by Belgian cartoonist Morris in 1946. The stories are filled with humorous elements parodying the Western genre. It is one of Europe's best-known and best-selling comic book series and has been translated into twenty-three languages.
2 The Dutch term '*wiskunde*' (mathematics) literally says 'art of erasing'/the art of cutting (as in Microsoft's Word, that is).
3 Schiller (2016 [1794]).
4 Silvio (1985).
5 Plant (2012).
6 In the song of French singer France Galle: '*Ella, elle l'a*', she has 'it': the small a object (-cause of desire) see later notes.

Chapter 7

Return to Freud

The Earliest Freud

Of course, Mark Solms was already a leading figure in the book I edited with Bazan. Indeed, partly due to the steep rise of his neuropsychoanalysis since then, he has become one of the leading figures in the wider psychoanalytic world. As recently as 2018, his article on *The scientific standing of psychoanalysis* was the most read in the international (online) edition of the *British Journal of Psychiatry*. The fact that, after James Strachey, he has been charged with editing a revised *Standard Edition* of Freud's four neurological and twenty-four psychological works provides evidence of his standing.[1] Suppose now and again he may come off a bit stilted. This extraordinary knowledge of Freud's oeuvre (in its original German version – Solms is Namibian by birth) may be a mitigating circumstance. Above all, however, this assertive style is based on decades of (neuro- and other) scientific research.

The occasion for writing this book was the publication of two of his books: *Clinical Studies in Neuropsychoanalysis Revisited*, which he edited with Christian Salas and Oliver Turnbull, in which Bazan represents the Lacanian approach. Second, Solms' *The Hidden Spring. A Journey to the Source of Consciousness*.[2] The first book harks back to a first edition[3] that he wrote with his then-wife, in which he integrated the clinical–anatomical with a psychoanalytic approach in patients and which needed an update after twenty years. In the second book, Solms aspires nothing less than to solve *the hard problem of consciousness*.[4] Cognitive science can analyse and reconstruct many functions, but how and why does something like subjective experience arise? Behold this so-called 'hard' problem. Solms adds Karl Friston's free energy principle from elementary physics and computational neuroscience to a more comprehensive interpretation of homeostasis from affective neuroscience. This leap forward will be discussed later. This was followed rapidly by three articles in which he successively revised Freud's *Project*, his drive theory and the Oedipus complex. It seemed an excellent opportunity to closely examine more than two decades of neuropsychoanalysis and comment here and there.

I made it explicit in my prologue that Freud and Jacques Lacan are the two most critical psychoanalytical authors to me. Lacan is known for his famous return to/'*retour à Freud*'.[5] In doing so, he set himself apart from Ego-psychology[6]

DOI: 10.4324/9781003394358-7

(from which, in his view, all psychoanalytic essence had disappeared) and returned to the early Freud of dream interpretation, the joke and a slip of the tongue, when the unconscious is still central and conceived of as primarily textual. As shown, Solms' turn is also a return to Freud, but to the *earliest* (neuroscientific) Freud. In his own words, Solms wants to finish nothing less than Freud's 1895 *Project for a Scientific Psychology*. Prophetically, in this text, Freud was already talking about homeostasis and the pursuit of minimal arousal as the default mode of mental functioning. Because of insufficient technological research resources, Freud let it slip in 1896 with pain in his heart. Because it was not published until 1950, Freud's neuroscientific activities also remained in the shadow of his later theorisation for a long time.

Solms recalls innumerable times that Freud worked as a neurologist for twenty years before leaving Vienna University for his private practice because of the lack of career opportunities there. He did have about two hundred neurological publications to his name.[7] Starting with the eels, he became a world authority on *cerebral palsy* in children, and his text on the conceptual framework of aphasias remains relevant today.[8] His patient population in the *Berggasse* compelled him to understand hysteria better, and hypnosis led him to unconscious psychological causation alias psychogenesis. In correspondence/transference with Wilhelm Fliess, he undertook a self-analysis (not least of his dreams) and would henceforth develop an entirely independent (meta-)psychological theory. Freud did continue to consider it necessary for (neuro-)biology to support the provisional assumptions of psychoanalysis over time. For instance, he called biology a land of unlimited possibilities. According to him, we could expect it to give us the most surprising insights, and we could not predict what answers it would provide us with several decades later. In his own words, they might undermine the whole artificial structure of his hypotheses.[9] But first, let us return for a moment to what Freud argued about.

Energy and Drive

In 1895, Freud wrote his *Project* in three weeks. In it, he tried to ground his later psychoanalysis in a (natural) scientific psychology. In retrospect, however, he called this ambition 'a kind of mistake'.[10] Following the affect/trauma model of his *Neurotica*, he replaced neuropsychology with metapsychology in the seventh chapter of his *The Interpretation of Dreams*.[11] However, he was (auto-) critical of this endeavour also. For instance, he called his drive theory 'drive mythology'[12] and his reflections on the primal horde a scientific myth.[13]

Today, things like the economic point of view and the drive have all but disappeared from psychoanalysis.[14] Nevertheless, energy was very much present in Freud's *Project*.[15] For example, in this text, he talks about the principle of neuronal inertia, where neurons strive to discharge completely.[16] This principle is supposed to determine the unconscious's primary process and free energy circulation. The pleasure principle is also an economic/energetic principle. It is primarily determined by the pursuit of reducing or avoiding unpleasure rather than by the pursuit of pleasure. In this sense, our drives are caused more by an excess than a lack of excitation.[17]

However, there remains much ambiguity: what does Freud mean by the pleasure principle? A striving for zero, for as low as possible or for constant tension? Do the former two determine the unconscious and primary process on the one hand and the latter the preconscious and conscious on the other? Do the later death and life drives aim for zero and constancy, respectively? Is the former entropic (aiming at dissolution) and the latter negentropic (aiming at binding)? In any case, there are two *kinds of* excitations (one of them the sexual) to which the organism is exposed and which it must get rid of according to the constancy principle, which will cha-racterise the Ego's functioning from the later structural model onward. After the pleasure principle settles, the reality principle only comes into being through lear-ning from experience. The initially free energy is thereby bound up in the secon-dary process of the preconscious and the conscious.[18] This more realistic secondary process thinking characterises the executive control systems of the frontal cortex.[19] The reality principle prevailing there ensures that we achieve goals or satisfaction. On the other hand, the pleasure principle continues to prevail in several psychic activities, including fantasy and dreaming.

The unconscious from Freud's first topical model was the repressed, while in the later structural model, the Id represents the vast and chaotic reservoir of drive energies.[20] The same principles prevail in the topical unconscious: the primary pro-cess, a complex organisation, and layered drives.[21] In this model, the repressed forms a compartment. It is separated from the Ego by the repression barrier and communicates with the Id.[22] The Id opens at the bottom to the somatic.[23] It, there-fore, lends itself more to a biologist or naturalising interpretations than the initial (indeed rather semiotically intelligible) unconscious.[24] Economically it involves a transformation from free to bound energy; topically, it involves preconscious and conscious vs unconscious; dynamically, in the reality principle, the drive energy comes to serve the Ego.

Freud discussed the concept of drive extensively in 1915 and 1920. In *Instincts and their vicissitudes*, it reads as follows: drive appears to us as a concept on the frontier between the mental and the somatic, as the psychical representative of the stimuli originating from within the organism and reaching the mind, as a measure of the demand made upon the reason for work in consequence of its connection with the body.[25] For Freud, the main objective of the drive is to discharge as quickly as possible excitations that reach the mind from within the body and thus keep the incessant somatic stimuli as low as possible. For him, the discharge of free energy defines our primary-process thinking.

While in his *Project*, he was still talking about the principle of neuronal inertia in which nerve cells reflexively discharge. After 1920 he introduced Barbara Low's Nirvana principle, according to which the nervous system gets rid of excitation as quickly as possible and pursues complete rest. In this view, the drive conforms to the Second Law of Thermodynamics. It is entropic. A somewhat uncomfortable conclusion, therefore, urged itself: pleasure results from the satisfaction of death drive. After a prior warning by Freud in the fourth chapter ('what follows is speculation'), this death drive as such is only introduced in *Beyond the Pleasure Principle*[26]... The death drive would then lead to tension zero.[27] We shall see that (from a biological point of view) Solms considers this death drive neuroscientific nonsense.[28] Once satisfied, all drives admittedly disappear under the radar. There is complete silence. But calling the biological ideal (in which all physical and emotional needs are satisfied), the death drive looks pretty contradictory to him. He also questions whether this death drive drills a hole, as it were, in the homeostatic. I will return to this towards this book's (more Lacanian) end.

In a variation of the pleasure principle, the constancy principle commands the maintenance of an energetic tonus that is kept as stable and constant as possible. Indeed, this tonus provides a store of bound and usable energy. It is utilised in the secondary process that compromises the primary process and the requirements of life or reality—the reality principle is a variation and upgrade of the pleasure principle. We come into the world with reflexes and instincts, but these need to be supplemented by learning from gratification and other experiences.[29] How it can satisfy the drive and through which objects are highly variable, with the object, in particular, being very much determined by life history.

Although Freud's drive was systematically translated as instinct by Strachey, they are different. Instinct is hereditary and appears in almost identical ways in all individuals of the same species. In contrast, the drive introduced by Freud in 1905 is highly variable. The object, in particular, is contingent. The final form the drive takes on depends on the drive's fate and the subject's history.[30] Following the model of hunger and love, first, Ego- or self-preservative drives are distinguished from sexual drives; later comes another drive-pair: the life and death drives,[31] love and hate. Note that Freud speaks of the drives as mythical beings, incredible in their indeterminacy.[32] From the beginning, the self-preservative drives are directed towards objects in reality; after all, they need to get satisfied. On the other hand, the connection between sexuality and phantasm is so essential that realism always remains more controversial here. This is abundantly clear from clinical practice. Self-preservation and realism go together, while sexuality remains more characterised by wish fulfilment.

Helicopter View

Solms' neuropsychoanalysis has already undergone quite a development since its conception.[33] Solms' initial clinical studies were based on a limited number of patients with focal brain damage treated through psychoanalytic therapy for only a few sessions by Solms and his ex-partner.[34] They still needed to reflect on the drastic influence that Jaak Panksepp's affective neuroscience would exert on the neuropsychoanalytic landscape.[35] This influence only gradually became noticeable throughout Solms' publications, culminating in his revolutionary article on *The Conscious Id*.[36]

Antonio Damasio had already made an impassioned plea in 1994 in *Descartes' Error* for more recognition of affect in cognitive science (that had begun to boom since the 1980s).[37] In it, he equated feelings with the registration of bodily states, where pleasant and unpleasant feelings are respectively related to increases or decreases in chances of survival or reproduction. According to Damasio, this is *why we have feelings at all.* Panksepp's findings confirmed his views.[38] Moreover, feelings refer to the inner body and brain states related to instinctive emotional systems such as attachment, anger or play.[39] By descending, like Panksepp, to the subcortical level, Damasio recognised that elementary forms of consciousness were much more primitive than first thought. Only belatedly would Solms join these reasonings.[40]

Following Antonio Damasio,[41] Solms did eventually come across homeostasis. It underlies consciousness as a biological principle, and via this homeostasis, as a negentropic principle, he arrived (after Panksepp and Damasio) at his third Great Inspirer: Karl Friston. His concepts of *predictive coding* and the *free energy principle*[42] allowed him to integrate the biology of homeostasis with the physics of entropy/uncertainty. I quote Solms[43] on the Eureka mood this gave him. 'When we came to that, I experienced something similar to what happened to Freud more than a century before, when he wrote to Wilhelm Fliess on 20 October 1895': *'Everything seemed to fit together, the gears were in mesh, the thing gave one the impression that it was really a machine and would soon run of itself... Of course, I cannot contain myself with delight'.*[44] Homeostasis, then, seemed to be able to explain the source of consciousness itself! The recognition of the importance of (the neurophysiology of) reconsolidation in learning and memory processes led to the further grounding of the method of psychoanalytic therapy, even in patients where there is no neurological problem.[45] Repressed desires are henceforth understood as prematurely automated predictions that therefore fail. This error leads to anxiety/free and unfettered energy and thus to the return, omnipresent in psychopathology, of what was repressed. Above all, recognising the free energy principle led to a different understanding of consciousness per se. Solms, therefore, makes a strong case for having solved the hard problem of consciousness with it. He, therefore, calls *The Hidden Source* the apotheosis of his life's work: a personal attempt to complete Freud's *Project for a Scientific Psychology*.[46] This is elaborated in a revision of Freud's original text, which is indeed updated, as it were, sentence by sentence, according to recent neuroscientific insights.[47] Solms also recently subjected the drive theory and the Oedipus complex to a thorough revision.[48]

Solms' Project

Again Antonio Damasio had put Phineas Gage, among others, on the stage in his *Descartes' Error*. In the summer of 1848, this unfortunate *rail worker* received a steel rod shot through the head, but mere minutes later, he was again going, standing and speaking. He retained almost normal functioning in perception, memory, language and intelligence. But Gage was no longer Gage. He disregarded social conventions, cursed like a sailor, lied, dismissed advice and was highly impulsive. The consequences were disastrous, and he became an attraction in a circus. Drawing on research from a dozen patients with similar brain injuries, Damasio concludes that to be cartesian/reasonable, we must be able to listen to our bodies and the feelings they express. Emotions play a key role in our practical reasoning. They are necessary to go over our options, weigh our choices and make decisions. Well, Solms has his project starting from a Phineas Gage incident from his personal life, namely his brother Lee's tragic accident. He fell off a roof and suffered a brain injury while their parents had gone yachting. Afterwards, he (like Gage) had changed most in character. Young Mark had the greatest difficulty in placing and understanding this. He relates the fact that he later went on to study neuropsychology to this drama. After all, the neuroscience of the time appeared to focus exclusively on cognitive cortical information processing and not on the *sentient mind.* Solms was 'displeased'.[49] He found a like-mind in neurologist and best-selling author Oliver Sacks. He repeatedly quotes his statement: '*Neuropsychology is admirable, but it excludes the psyche... It is precisely the subject, the living I, which is excluded from* neurology'.[50] As is now well known, with forty-six years of psychoanalysis with Leonard Shengold, Sacks is probably the world record holder for long-term psychoanalysis.[51] He delved into the inner world of his imaginative neurological patients with his *single case studies*. Most famous (by the book's title of the same name) is perhaps *The Man Who Mistook his Wife for a Hat.*

The cognitive sciences that came to the fore at the end of the last century mainly took their inspiration from computer science. They also initially completely ignored emotional and motivational feeling states and the neural substrate underlying them (logical, chronological, phylogenetic *and* ontogenetic). In retrospect, a computer has language and memory, can perceive (fingerprints or face recognition) and make predictions using algorithms. Only it lacks consciousness and subjectivity to be understood as what it is/feels like to *be* a computer. Philosopher John Searle launched a famous thought experiment on this in 1980,[52] namely the Chinese Room. His conclusion: just because a computer acts like a human doesn't mean it feels (itself) like a human. Computers can easily beat humans in all sorts of cognitive respects, but they do not develop consciousness. If you ask the computer a question, it does not understand you; it just applies pre-programmed algorithms. Artificial intelligence made great strides in recent decades. Still, while computers can solve problems, they lack the affective motivations of *sentient* animals and the biological foundations in which our minds are grounded.[53] Again in a bold look, Solms today has formed a group of scientists around him who want to design an artificially intelligent robot with consciousness. In other words, not just a robot sapiens, but also a robot *sentiens*. In doing so, Solms follows the motto physicist Richard Feynman noted in his diary on 4 October 2019: *What I cannot create, I do not understand.*[54] Some people shudder at such samples of trans-humanist technology. Proponents feel it does not matter whether consciousness runs on carbon or silicon compounds. What would be so special about the flesh?[55] However, these are (only) opinions. After all, connoisseurs apply the principle of organismic invariance. It simply implies that two systems with the same sophisticated functional organisation will have qualitatively similar experiences.[56]

Solms became interested in psychoanalysis after a comparative literature seminar on the interpretation of dreams. Before that, he was sceptical of psychoanalysis, which was, after all considered (also at the South African University of Witwatersrand) a pseudoscience.[57] Traditionally primarily interested in his own and all of us human subjectivity, Solms took a five-year psychoanalytic course in London, where he immersed himself in Freudian and (post-)Kleinian thought in particular.[58] This was to give back a place to the (living) I in his neuroscientific research.

Clinical–Anatomical Method

In his research, Solms took further inspiration from the clinical–anatomical method of Broca, Charcot, Luria and partly Freud to investigate correlations between the mental and the neuronal.[59] Briefly and concisely, what neurological damage corresponds to what loss of mental function and vice versa? He does conceive of the localisation of mental function in specific brain parts as dynamic rather than static. For instance, Ellis and Solms[60] argue that (primarily cognitive) brain abilities are not innate but highly experience-dependent. Neuroplasticity is undetermined in the sense that connections are continuously formed and deformed.[61]

While no attention is usually paid (anymore) to the inner world of neurological patients (especially with cerebrovascular accidents or with brain tumours), Solms used with them the clinic of the ear, not the (medical) clinic of the gaze. Above all, he examined their stories and their dreams. In this sense, he put into practice the motto of French psychiatrist and psychoanalyst Juan-David Nasio:[62] The unconscious (even in neurological patients!) exists only for those who listen to it. Neuropsychologist by training, Solms will simultaneously follow in the footsteps of Freud and his mentor Ernst Brücke in taking up the thread of the Helmholtz School. These distanced themselves from a shadowy and immaterial life force and instead assumed that '*no other forces than the common physical and chemical ones are active within the organism*'.[63] In this view, consciousness cannot be a supernatural or extra-natural thing, but we should seek its origin within nature.

Especially after reading *The Conscious Id*[64] and a compilation of his most influential articles in *The Feeling Brain*,[65] I have become more convinced of Solms' particular neuropsychoanalytic added value. Psychoanalysis is not a technical discipline like dentistry: how do I place a filling? How do I treat a root canal? Its method and technique can only come about on the basis of a good/correct understanding of how our brain and mind essentially (do not) work. This is also why Freud's technical writings make up only a tiny fraction of a hundred pages or so in his more than eight thousand-page collected work. With his clinical–anatomical method, Solms constantly sought correlations between the brain and mind. He was one of the first to start listening psychoanalytically to neurological patients instead of reducing them to damaged and suffering objects. He increased the scientific and social relevance of discredited psychoanalysis by reinstating Freud's dream theory and introducing a different, more generally accessible language; he falsified Freud's localisation of conscious and unconscious because he placed consciousness convincingly subcortical and not cortical. He demonstrated these determinations through the famous argument of double dissociation, about which there is more below.

Solms makes the difference between the topical (conscious, preconscious, unconscious) and the structural (Id, Ego, Superego) models more transparent than ever. The unconscious is a representational and memory (and hence prediction!) system, and the Id is a drive system. While Freud distilled his drive theory from the psychoanalytic cure on the couch, Solms also connected to findings from animal research: *from the couch to the lab*.[66] Not only did he integrate cognitive and affective neuroscience into psychoanalytic theory and technique, he tried to finish Freud's *Project* in the light of recent neuroscientific findings, and last but not least, he tried to explain how and why phenomenal consciousness occurs.

Science has already stolen many miracles. Free after Max Weber, not only the outer world but also our inner world is gradually becoming increasingly disenchanted by it. After Freud, Solms also clarifies that scientific exploration of the mind can paradoxically increase enchantment too!

Solms' Dream

Freud quotes French moralist Saint-Just on several occasions: '*On revient toujours à ses premiers amours*'.[67] One always returns to one's first love. His neuroscientific investigation of dreams (evidently subjective phenomenon par excellence) has made Mark Solms a psychoanalytic celebrity.[68] The account of his evolving findings reads like a *whodunnit*, in which Solms, in turn, falsified Alan Hobson's activation-synthesis theory of dreams.

Freud's dream interpretation and psychoanalysis were, in a sense, same-born. The dream as a guardian of sleep, as a veiled fulfilment of a wish and as a *via regia*/royal road to the unconscious are equally fundamental tenets for psychoanalysis.[69] Now, due to the philosophical criticism of science by Grünbaum and Popper and the *ad hominem* criticisms that characterised Freud-bashing[70] psychoanalysis had fallen into disrepute after World War II. But the discovery of REM sleep further shook Freud's premises. It is also called paradoxical sleep because the sleeper's brain appears active during this phase. Put paradoxically, dreams are a consciousness that does not know it is conscious. With a clock's purely mechanical and rhythmic regularity, REM sleep occurs in humans and animals. Alan Hobson did neuroscience research on cats (which have a talent for/patent on sleep). REM sleep stopped after the lesion of their pons. The location of the dream seemed to be found. Still, Hobson said dreams were neither more nor less than the meaningless conglomeration of haphazard acetyl-cholinergic activity during REM sleep.[71] The visual cortex is randomly stimulated, and meaning is added to it, just as you can see all sorts of things in a cloud or Rorschach blot without any prior sense. REM sleep and dream, according to Hobson, were the objective and subjective flip sides of the same coin.

After presenting his activation-synthesis theory[72] on the dream, two-thirds of the *American Psychiatric Association* turned away from the cornerstone of psychoanalysis in 1976: Freud's dream theory.

For his PhD thesis, Mark Solms[73] conducted research over five years on three hundred and sixty-one brain-damaged patients whom (unlike cats) he could *question*. He focused not on mental abilities such as perception, memory or language but on their dreams.[74] He came to (also for him) surprising and unexpected conclusions. In neuroscientific research, Hans-Lukas Teuber[75] developed the paradigm of double dissociation. This states that it involves two distinct neuropsychological functions when function A is lost due to damage to structure X but not due to damage to structure Y and when function B is lost due to damage to structure Y but not due to damage to structure X. (Here, A is the dream and B is REM sleep and X is the midbrain and Y is the pons). Well, such double dissociation appeared to falsify Hobson's conclusions. Briefly, REM sleep and dreams are independent of each other. Shutting down the neurological *pathways* of one leaves the other function intact in both directions.

Solms' analysis of the data led to the hypothesis that the *pathway* of the dream originates in the ventral tegmental area of the midbrain, runs through the pleasure nucleus/*nucleus accumbens* via the white pathways of the basal forebrain and then through the mesocortical and mesolimbic systems. It is also known as the brain's motivational circuitry: it prompts goal-directed behaviour and pleasurable interaction with the outside world.[76] The *pathway* that causes dreams is precisely that of Panksepp's[77] SEEKING system: the most energetic, exploring and searching behaviour also causes our dreams.[78] Solms notes laconically that the fact that (not only wet) dreams involve erection was systematically ignored.[79]

That SEEKING plays a role in the dream was already apparent from some famous historical examples. I am thinking, for instance, of three dreams Descartes had on the night of 10 November 1619 in which his entire philosophy found its foreshadowing.[80] To Friedrich Kekulé's benzene ring, which he discovered after seeing a snake biting its tail in a dream.[81] Or to the famous poem *Kubla Khan*, which the British Romantic poet Samuel Coleridge jotted down in one gulp immediately after waking up and then subtitled *A Vision in a Dream*.[82]

Dream images do not appear to be the product of direct activation of the visual zones but rather of regression of action intentions that are motor blocked to higher integration centres.[83] Thus, Solms presents a model that corresponds with Freud's dream theory in many respects. His research was subsequently confirmed by, for example, Yu[84] and Colace.[85] The latter provides nomothetic evidence that the dream contains a compromise between desires and moral constraints. Childhood dreams change with the installation of the Superego around the age of five. Before, they are manifestly wish-fulfilling; only afterwards, they undergo distortions as if gratification collides with internal obstacles.

When Solms consulted the earlier literature surrounding frontal lobotomy (an operation in the same neuroanatomical zone) performed on thousands of patients against the positive symptoms of psychosis, this operation was found to have three effects: delusions and hallucinations reduced or disappeared, patients ended up in an a-motivational state and last but not least: they no longer dreamed.[86] At the 2006 biennial of *The Science of Consciousness Congress* in Tucson, Arizona, thirty years after the first one, a vote was taken among the participants. This time, two-thirds were convinced of the validity of Freud's dream theory.[87] Psychoanalysis was back in town. Many thanks for that, Mark.

Endnotes

1 Solms (2021b).
2 Salas, Turnbull, and Solms (2021).
3 Solms (2021d).
4 Kaplan-Solms and Solms (2000).
5 Chalmers (1995a, 1995b). The hard problem is how and why we can have qualia, defined as 'individual instances of subjective, conscious experience'.
6 Masson (2019).
7 Roughly until the Second World War, Ego-psychology was dominant in American psychoanalysis with figures like Heinz Hartmann, Ernst Kris and Rudolph Löwenstein. It leaned heavily towards psychiatry and behavioural therapy, conceived of the Ego as autonomous and adaptive, and led to techniques Lacan reportedly somewhat disparagingly called orthopaedics of the soul. Löwenstein was Lacan's analyst.
8 Solms and Saling (1986, 1990). Solms repeatedly insists on the neurological antecedents of Freud, while the latter introduced the term psychoanalysis only later. The work of Freud (as well as that of Lacan) consists of several eras, and it is not so easy to declare this or that era as 'true' psychoanalysis. Psychoanalysis is an evolving science; later insights do not (entirely) erase earlier ones but complement them. They often merely nuance or amend earlier formulations.
9 Solms (1998).
10 How Freud's friend and correspondent Wilhelm Fliess also functioned as a transference figure is nicely shown in Didier Anzieu's book (1975).
11 Freud (1920a, p. 183, 1940b, p. 202).
12 Letter to Fliess, dated 29/11/1895, in Freud (1950b, p. 134).
13 Freud (1900a, 1900b).
14 Freud (1933a, p. 157, 1933b, p. 185).
15 Freud (1921c, p. 285, 1921d, p. 135).
16 Solms (2021e, p. 1036).
17 'Though we have no means of measuring it' (Freud 1894, p. 60) in Solms (2021e, p. 1037).
18 Laplanche and Pontalis (1967, p. 329).
19 Freud (1900a, p. 600, 1900b, p. 629).
20 In a rudimentary Bionian (1962) terminology, an energetic force (♂) is taken up and processed by the psychic container (♀).
21 Solms and Turnbull (2002).
22 Freud (1923b, pp. 63–67, notes 1 and 46).
23 Freud (1933a, pp. 73–74; 1933b, pp. 5–6).
24 Laplanche and Pontalis (1967, p. 58).
25 Freud (1915b, pp. 121–122).
26 Freud (1920b, p. 63).
27 Freud (1920a, pp. 160, 341).
28 When Lacan begins to develop his Trinity of imaginary, symbolic and real (chronologically), he argues that the death drive is simply the fundamental tendency of the symbolic order to produce repetition. 'The death drive is only the mask of the symbolic

order' (1988b, p. 326). Lacan's death drive must be distinguished from the biological drive to return to the inanimate/inorganic. It is firmly articulated with culture (1992, pp. 211–212). Lacan's concept of the drive is -more generally- removed from the realm of biology. Drives differ from biological needs in that they can never be satisfied. They do not aim at an object but circle it. The purpose of the drive is not to reach a final destination but to follow its aim (Lacan 1981b, p. 168). *Jouissance*/enjoyment resides in the repetitive movement of this closed circuit. See later in the book.

29   Solms (2018b, 2018c).
30   Freud (1915e, 1915f).
31   I quote Freud on the fundamental importance psychoanalysis attributes to the *sexual* drive (1917, p. 138): 'Unintelligent opposition accuses us of one-sidedness in our estimate of the sexual instincts. "Human beings have other interests besides sexual ones", they say. We have not forgotten or denied this for a moment [hence Freud's self-preservation drives, MK]. Our one-sidedness is like that of the chemist, who traces all compounds back to the force of chemical attraction. He is not on that account denying the force of gravity; he leaves that to the physicist to deal with'. Later on in Freud's work, there is a fundamental opposition between life drives (Eros), conceived of as a tendency towards cohesion and unity, and the death drives (Thanatos), undoing connections and destroying things. These life and death drives are never found in a pure state. They are always mixed/fused in differing proportions. Were it not for this fusion with erotism, the death drive would elude our perceptions since it is mute/silent (Freud 1930, p. 120).
32   Freud (1933a, p. 95).
33   Solms and Turnbull (2011), Balchin et al. (2019).
34   Kaplan-Solms and Solms (2000).
35   Panksepp and Solms (2012), Solms and Panksepp (2012).
36   Solms (2013a).
37   Solms (2021d, p. 62).
38   Panksepp (1998).
39   Damasio (2018), Solms (2018a).
40   Solms and Panksepp (2012).
41   Damasio (1994, 1999).
42   Solms and Friston (2018), Solms (2019a).
43   Solms (2019a, note 38, own transl.).
44   Letter to Fliess, dated 20/10/1895, in Freud (1950a [1892–1899]).
45   Solms (2015a) and see further.
46   Solms (2017a, 2018b, 2018c).
47   Solms (2021d, p. 10).
48   Solms (2020).
49   Solms (2021f).
50   Salas, Turnbull, and Solms (2021, p. 13).
51   Sacks (1984, p. 164).
52   Roth (2015).
53   Searle (1980) see https://plato.stanford.edu/entries/chinese-room/
54   Lauwaert (2021).
55   Feynman (2019).
56   I quote David Chalmers (2022, p. 49) himself in this regard: I think the safest way to do it is to gradually replace a bit of my brain, by, say, replace some neurons by silicon chips, replace 1 per cent of my brain, 5 per cent of my brain, 10 per cent of my brain, 20 per cent, 50 per cent, till eventually 100 per cent of your brain has been replaced by silicon chips. Ideally, you could stay conscious throughout this process, so I could say: 'Okay, I am still here. I am still experiencing this'. If there was a continuous chain of consciousness from the biological brain to the uploaded brain, then I think there is a pretty good case that would still be me'.

57 Solms (2021d, p. 325).
58 Solms (2021d, p. 44).
59 I return to this when I discuss his clinical work.
60 Kaplan-Solms and Solms (2000), Solms (2000b).
61 Ellis and Solms (2018).
62 Ansermet and Magistretti (2007).
63 Nasio (1992).
64 Du Bois-Reymond (1918).
65 Solms (2013a).
66 Cited in Freud (1905a, p. 36, 1905b, p. 152, 1913a, p. 273, 1913b, p. 184).
67 Solms (2015b).
68 Solms and Zellner (2012).
69 Solms (1991, 1997, 2000a, 2001, 2021a).
70 Freud (1900a, 1900b).
71 The term Freud-bashing refers to various *ad hominem* criticisms of Freud: that he experimented with cocaine (its introduction as a painkiller was snatched from him by a colleague), that he allegedly had an extramarital affair with his sister-in-law, that he embellished case studies, that he (also) made non-analytical interventions and so on. As if the (even minor) human missteps of Picasso or Einstein would detract any value from their artistic or scientific contributions.
72 Solms (1997, 2000a).
73 Hobson and Mc Carly (1977).
74 Solms (2021, p. 33).
75 Solms (1997).
76 Davies (2010).
77 See further in Panksepp (1998).
78 Solms (2021d, p. 40).
79 Ibid., p. 28.
80 Withers (2008).
81 Rocke (2010).
82 Coleridge (1816).
83 Dreams and other expressions of primary-process thinking are meaningful, wish-fulfilling results of the loss of frontal executive control of mesocortical and mesolimbic SEEKING systems (Solms and Turnbull 2002).
84 Yu (2001a, 2001b).
85 Colace (2012).
86 Solms (2021d, p. 38).
87 Ibid., p. 48.

Chapter 8

Interlude

An Atlas with Burnout

Sam is an athletic fifty-something with a lot of flower power. He is an only child. His mother was in education. She always wants to do the right thing for everyone and is described as over-protective. 'Over' because sometimes he finds her a little bit overbearing. All in all, she was somewhat of a hindrance to his development. Father is a retired labourer. Sam looked up to his father very much as a boy because he was so handy and could repair anything. Sam says he was reasonably happy during the first years of his life. However, the father's alcohol abuse caused many tensions and conflicts at home. When drinking, he was physically aggressive and threatening and sometimes injured his mother. On several occasions, she had to flee the house with Sam. Sam tried to understand and mediate, feeling constantly caught between his parents. He always felt different from his peers. After all, he had a secret. He had something to hide. Everything was covered up (in large part due to pressure from his mother). She insisted on keeping up appearances. For his part, Sam felt that everything was wrong at home. He never thought he belonged anywhere and anxiously tried to meet everyone's expectations. His studies came second. His main job was to guard and keep the peace at home. Although an outstanding student, he obtained (only) a bachelor's degree. He feels he has not lived up to his full potential. He worked for a company for a long time but quit because he experienced a lack of confirmation there. 'I expected too much; I want appreciation and impact'.

Since then, he has worked as a municipal clerk. He lived with his parents for a long time. He would go out a lot and drink excessively. Easily a crate of Belgian lager a day. He quotes the advertising slogan: 'Men know why'. He wrecked several cars. He only gained sexual experience, thanks to paid love. Relationally, he was in an amorous relationship with a prostitute for a long time. She was reportedly a victim of human trafficking for sexual exploitation and was terrorised by a pimp. He had emotionally profound conversations with her and forged plans to rescue her from the clutches of bad men. Although she received him scantily dressed and ready for sex, he was not so interested in sexual contact. Instead, he felt an ardent platonic infatuation that made him laud her innocence despite glaring evidence to the contrary. He offered her financial support and considered kidnapping and taking her and all her belongings to a safe place. One does not have to be Sigmund

DOI: 10.4324/9781003394358-8

Freud to understand that this is an idealising maternal fixation. A romantic love purged of sensual components goes hand in hand with fantasies of chivalry and rescue, eliminating the evil father/rival. Over the years, Sam has come to consult me a few times. He has a few sessions during these periods, but each time quickly breaks off treatment. Although he is very docile towards me, he also has much pent-up anger. He does not want me to say very much and considers keeping his world to himself 'normal'.

After a few years of absence, he came looking for me again. He had remained sober all this time. In the meantime, he had lived alone, and for several years, he had had an affair with a much younger female colleague who still lived with her parents. They often went out or travelled. His girlfriend seemed to have all sorts of anxieties and complexes. She also struggled with depression. De facto, he quickly became more of a support system than a partner. He took her from one counselling service to another. At work, he secured a permanent contract for himself, but his supervisor played a 'dirty trick' on him. Although he had passed specific exams and been promised a promotion, through nepotism, a competitor landed the post he had aspired to. His girlfriend also moved up the ladder, and although less qualified, her salary was now much higher than his. All this frustrates him greatly. 'Others move up, and I am stuck in my place'.

I have sketched his background to outline another aspect of his problems. He spent many a session discussing social issues. Especially the neoliberal altar of More, Faster and Better. How a capitalist juggernaut is crushing the little man in particular. How we perish on a crazy economic treadmill. How we are exploiting Mother Earth and destroying it. He spent much of his spare time in an alternative community where sustainable conservation and ecological horticulture were high on the agenda. There he met like-minded people who joined hands (literally, too) in an atmosphere of emotional openness. He also devoured all sorts of books debunking progress and advocating replacing patriarchal madness with a society organised on a more egalitarian basis. In each case, he is very passionate in his argument but equally frustrated that he is, like David, who repeatedly loses to Goliath. He is constantly on the move, running from place to place to help everyone. Meanwhile, he complains that he is taking little care of himself. He wants to go on a trip, go for a walk by the sea, and have a nice, sumptuous meal at a restaurant but has yet to get around to it. He is tired and wonders where all this is leading to. He is alone and lacks a life companion.

We don't remember ever wanting to be the One and Only for one or both of our parents, and to this end, wanting to eliminate our competitors. These symbolic-imaginary variations on themes resonate with stereotypes associated with the Oedipus complex. Sam first looked for mythological references when I compared him to an Atlas with burnout. He came up with the Battle of the Titans. Only after many decades of drinking and drowning his feelings is he finally now analysing this battle once and for all.

Chapter 9

The Drive on the Rise

Charles Darwin

To discuss integrating affective neuroscience into psychoanalysis, I must first refer to Charles Darwin.[1] In *On the Origin of Species* from 1859, he clearly states that the difference between humans and animals is gradual/dimensional and not categorical ('one of degree and not of kind').[2] We further read in the final chapter that psychology will be placed on a new foundation, that of the necessary acquisition of all mental powers and faculties through gradual transition'.[3] On several occasions, he quotes the motto: *Natura non facit saltum (*nature makes no leaps). In his *An Outline of Psychoanalysis*, Freud also says that this general (Id/Ego/Superego or structural M.K.) scheme of the psychic apparatus will also be able to be applied to the higher psychically similar animals to man. Wherever, as in humans, a relatively long period of filial dependence has existed, one can postulate a Superego. According to Freud, separating Ego and Id is an inescapable hypothesis.

Darwin, as we know, occupied a central place in Freud's mind (and his London headquarters). In later books such as *The Descent of Man* (1871) and *The Expression of Emotions in Man and Animals* (1872), Darwin sheds additional light on the evolution of humans' emotional and cognitive faculties in common with other mammals. Four characteristics of homo sapiens (tool use, language, aesthetic sense and religion) are present in rudimentary form in non-human animals. Even morality is taken to be a result of evolution. In *The Descent of Man*, Darwin writes that only our innate bias and arrogance (that led our ancestors to declare that they were descended from demigods) make us object to this conclusion.[4] According to mainstream evolutionary theory, we should assume that our cognitive and emotional faculties are inherited from our evolutionary ancestors. Such abilities are homologous. They must be distinguished from analogous traits. These have a (more or less) joint appearance and a (more or less) common function but no shared genealogical ancestry. For example, the form of a dolphin is analogous to that of a fish but homologous to that of a whale.

I apologise for referring to Darwin at some length here. Many humanists continue to need help with his evolutionary theory. With the vertebrates, however, we have in common a 525-million-year-old brain structure and physiology that makes

DOI: 10.4324/9781003394358-9

us aware of pleasure and unpleasure in a rudimentary way, so we experience attraction and repulsion phenomena, respectively. This pleasure principle has been refined and has diversified in mammals into very different forms of pleasure and unpleasure that determine our actions. Here, the brain mechanisms are about 200 million years old. We play, copulate, fight, flee, and are sensitive to care, separation, etc. Less than a million years ago, our forehead and brain grew. This prefrontal lobe allows us to inhibit (and not blindly follow our instincts), act provisionally only within the virtual reality of our head (in other words, think) and interact with the world more flexibly and in adapted ways.

Jaak Panksepp

Jaak Panksepp,[5] highly regarded by Solms, fits entirely in the Darwinian tracks that have been outlined. In 2007, he became world-famous in wider circles for recording the high-frequency sound (55 kilohertz) of rats laughing,[6] a sound inaudible to humans because its frequency is too high. Still, fortunately, some of his findings are more relevant to psychoanalysis. He conducted countless experiments (especially in rodents) by electrically or chemically stimulating certain brain regions and studying the resulting behaviour.[7] Panksepp links rat and human brains through a nested brain hierarchy concept.[8] Humans date back to the Pleistocene, but, as mentioned before, the emotional part of our brain goes back much further, namely to the time when mammals evolved away from reptiles. Primary emotional processes in the deepest subcortical structures originate from that time. Above that is a layer of secondary processes where the basal ganglia act as stations and where feelings are enriched by learning: connecting perceptions with corresponding feelings. Above that, the neocortex provides higher cognitive processes that process life events. Our thinking is fuelled by memory and knowledge gained from physically and socially complex living conditions.

If we look at the clinic, successive editions of the *Diagnostic and Statistical Manual of Mental Disorders* (DSM for short) are well known to be full of emotions running amok. Emotions are powerful, even overwhelming forces. As soon as the individual registers them, they become feelings, and psychiatrists are, in a sense, doctors for these feelings. Patients suffer from them; they do not understand or want to get rid of them as quickly as possible. Pharmacotherapy can often be highly effective and efficient, but we are left (maybe 'better' but) no wiser for it.[9] Better understanding requires *psychotherapy*. Not behavioural therapy because it wants to focus precisely on observable behaviour. For it, the black box was allowed to remain closed. For the leading behaviourists Thorndike, Pavlov, Watson, and Skinner, (un-)learning is just the coupling of stimuli and responses.

I refer to an infamous statement by Skinner: emotions are but the fictional causes to which we attribute our problems.[10] Cognitive science (that is to say, cognitive behavioural therapy) also ignores the idiosyncrasy of feelings. If they are wrong, we should try/learn to replace them with the 'right' ones. But emotions are (phylogenetically and ontogenetically) ancient. They don't just allow themselves to be tamed. Feelings have both a reason and a right to exist.[11] They are useful. They contribute to our survival. That is simple evolutionary theory.

According to Edward Thorndike,[12] our minds are governed by the law of effect: behaviour that is always followed by reward increases, and that which is followed by punishment decreases. This process of learning by experience is called conditioning. Animals learn not by thinking but by making mistakes. We will see that Solms corrects Thorndike with just one letter: opposite the law of effect, he places the law of *affect,* which is not different from Freud's law of the pleasure principle. We animals repeat behaviour that makes us feel good, and we abandon behaviour that triggers unpleasant feelings.[13] According to Solms, affect-driven voluntary behaviour gives us a substantial adaptive advantage over involuntary behaviour: it frees us from the straitjacket of automaticity. It enables us to survive in unexpected situations.[14]

The Layered Brain

Before proceeding, I will make a rough sketch for the layman.[15] Like on horseback, the brain sits like a giant walnut on the brain stem. It represents about three per cent of our body weight but consumes about twenty-five per cent of our energy. From bottom to top, the spinal cord passes into the extended medulla or *medulla oblongata*, the *pons* and the midbrain. At the back of the brainstem is the *cerebellum*. Above it is the occipital lobe (mainly visually oriented); further forward on both sides, the parietal lobe (predominantly sensory oriented); above the ear, the temporal lobe (oriented primarily for hearing and memory) and in the front, the frontal cortex (mainly motor and oriented towards (to be thought of as trial action) thinking and judgement). Roughly speaking, the so-called limbic system is between the brainstem and cortex, as the headquarters of our emotionality. The brain consists of two hemispheres connected by white matter through the *corpus callosum*. There is lateralisation: each hemisphere places its specific emphases.

The brain and mind can be divided roughly into two essential parts.[16] First, there is the affective/instinctive core. Second (chronologically) is the inhibitory/cognitive/symbolic upper layer.[17] The latter is decisively influenced by and fundamentally also serves the first layer. We will see that, according to Solms, they correlate primarily with the psychoanalytic distinction between the Id on the one hand and the Ego/Superego on the other.[18]

The affective/instinctive layer contains the circuits that mediate the drives, instincts and primary emotions we have in common with all other mammals. They drive us to satisfy our needs. The blind watchmaker of evolution designed our basic emotions for survival and procreation. We don't have to learn them. They activate us in an involuntary and highly physical way. Our regulatory functions allow us to inhibit our impulses, creating the necessary mental space to plan our behaviour. We learn from positive and negative experiences. We possess thinking skills and imagination, allowing us to invent alternatives and create things/possibilities that did not yet exist. These latter processes are more random, more abstract and less embodied. Moreover, they are intertwined with our analogue and digital, semiotic and symbolic language learning.[19]

Emotional responses are mainly regulated by the collection of subcortical brain structures called the limbic system. It consists of the *hypothalamus*, which determines bodily reactions such as heart rhythm or perspiration, and the *amygdala*, which orchestrates our initial emotional responses. In much psychopathology, the *amygdala* and *hypothalamus* are constantly overactive, and many substances the limbic system uses are out of balance.[20] The brain's dopamine-reward system regulates pleasure from food, sex or drugs. It consists of the dopamine-producing neurons of the *substantia nigra*, which extend deep into the *hippocampus*, *amygdala* and *striatum* (all belonging to the limbic system).[21] The *hippocampus* is involved in declarative memory, the *amygdala* regulates primary emotions, and the *striatum* plays a key role in developing habits. The *cerebellum*, then, is involved in almost all activities/layers of our brain.

All mammals have the same brain infrastructure for primary drives and instincts. We have the same needs, the same species-specific ways of imagining these needs and similar forms of interacting with the environment to satisfy needs and ward off dangers. All mammals can register their internal and external bodies and the outside world, allowing them to navigate according to their needs. All possess some ability to inhibit behaviour and learn on multiple levels. They differ among themselves mainly in the size and proportion of the association cortex. This cortex integrates the raw material of primary sensory and motor signals, leading to representations of a higher/more abstract order. It increases as we ascend the evolutionary bush.

Great apes have more extraordinary (cap-)abilities than rats. Primatological figureheads like Jane Goodall or Frans de Waal[22] repeatedly contrast anthropomorphism with '*anthropodenial*'. We need not ascribe human characteristics to animals, nor should we deny our (sometimes very close) kinship. Despite our cultural and technical achievements, we have ninety-five per cent of our emotional and social dispositions in common with primates. For that matter, do our technical ingenuity and cultural achievements make such a big difference? In an analogy: Narcissus remains the same whether he is fascinated by his reflection in the water or by that of a selfie. Even (or even a fortiori) in times of in vitro fertilisation, an Oedipus can indulge in incest or parricide entirely unknowingly. Our neighbours, the chimpanzees and gorillas, have the most developed cognitive potential. They have *mirror-self recognition*. Even though the sight of their mirror image does not cause jubilation or fascination as it does for the still fragmentary human child. They can, however, manipulate or feign things like symbols.[23] There is also evidence for some rudimentary *theory of mind*.[24] Like many other animals, great apes dream and even use *American Sign Language* while dreaming.[25]

Only humans constantly remember specific events and have images of the future.[26] You can call it imagination, daydreaming, fantasy, autobiographical memory or *mental time travel*. They are mainly realised in the association cortex, particularly in the *default mode network*. Neuroanatomically, the default mode network involves the lower parietal lobe and the anterior and posterior medial cortex.[27] People use symbols and can regulate their behaviour thanks to a highly complex integration of imagined or predicted outcomes. They can consider the perspectives of others and a wide variety of cues and adjust their behaviour accordingly.

The Drive on the Rise

According to emotion psychologist Paul Ekman,[28] human beings can have as many as ten thousand facial expressions thanks to their thirty-three facial muscles. Seven seem universally human and globally recognisable: fear, disgust, anger, joy, sadness, surprise and contempt. These are the primary, mainly genetically determined and evolutionarily older basic emotions. They can exist individually: after all, you can comfortably feel happy or angry alone. They need to be distinguished from secondary social emotions such as, for example, shame, shyness or guilt. These are complex, occur only within a social context and are related to the self and self-esteem. In contrast to basic emotions, they do not show themselves so quickly on a person's face.

In turn, Jaak Panksepp's affective neuroscience distinguishes between sensory, homeostatic and emotional affects. They correspond to what we commonly understand as reflexes, drives and instincts. Sensorial (exteroceptive) affects are surprise, pain and aversion. They are closely related to motor reflexes. Homeostatic affects are hunger, thirst, heat/cold, and breathlessness. These affects regulate the essential needs of the body. Freud called them drives: the source of his psychic energy, which was the driving force of the psychic mechanism. I mentioned it earlier: many psychoanalysts reject Freud's drive theory/the drive concept today.[29] On top of the drive are instincts, defined as unlearned behavioural responses towards the environment: breeding and nesting behaviour, migration of birds and other animals, hibernation, salmon swimming upstream and so on. A new-born mouse stiffens when confronted with a cat's hair, as does a field mouse when caught in the shadow of a bird of prey.[30] They don't have to learn this from mum and dad; this knowledge is pre-programmed through natural selection. We can inhibit it but not erase it.

Of particular psychoanalytic interest, of course, are emotional affects. They are rooted in seven emotional-instinctive neuronal and behavioural programmes mapped by Jaak Panksepp. They are written in capitals below because they are evolutionarily homologous circuits. They operate within the same brain structures, and their neuromodulators and receptors regulate each. They allow our emotional life to be carved at its joints. They are, as it were, natural kinds. They can be seen as innate tendencies to respond physically or behaviourally in adaptively beneficial ways to situations that present universal biological challenges.

The SEEKING system is the leading system and is considered most similar to Freud's libido.[31] The drive is the mental sensation of SEEKING: the urge to act to achieve a desired goal. It is without an object. In Panksepp's terms: '*a goad* without *a goal*'.[32] SEEKING, as it were, proactively seeks surprise or uncertainty, and this incentive hunger and sometimes the risky urge for discovery makes us more/better prepared to face the future. After all (paraphrasing a famous laconic remark by Wilfred Bion): life is full of surprises, most disagreeable. SEEKING drives one to explore the world, and it induces an exciting affect, from optimistic to enthusiastic, also caused by psychoactive substances such as cocaine and amphetamine. What is remarkable about SEEKING is that it can also come ON during our sleep, triggered by emerging needs or desires. Thus, it underlies the formation of dreams.[33] The other systems provide the SEEKING system with a goal. When their homeostatic equilibrium is reached, the SEEKING engages in so-called epistemic foraging. Once we have this luxury, we can indulge in discovery per se. It has the adaptive advantage of allowing us to minimise subsequent prediction errors.

The SEEKING system has no *pre-wired* notions of the object it is searching for. It primarily drives us to engage with the external world. It is the neurobiological basis of my favourite quote, usually attributed to American short-story writer Dorothy Parker. '*The only cure for boredom is curiosity; for curiosity, there is no cure*'. The SEEKING system must interact with the other systems to assign a value to the objects sought or found, and it must be able to 'save these interactions as experiences to learn from'.[34] SEEKING in itself has nothing to do with reward or pleasure. They are derived from the (opioid) LIKING system (that Kent Berridge put on the map). SEEKING involves appetite, understood as pleasure-anticipated arousal. Still, when gratification fails, there is frustration, and this system falls flat – comparisons with Freud's *Vorlust* or Lacanian enjoyment ('*jouissance*')[35] come to mind. I will return to this later on in connection with Ariane Bazan.

The SEEKING system underlies three primary emotional systems that support pro-social behaviour: LUST (sexuality), CARE (parental care) and PLAY (joyful social exercise).[36] These systems are pro-social because they appeal to others and promote positive connections. They are mediated by neurotransmitters such as opioids and dopamine, both of which lead to strong positive affect (warmth, simple pleasure with opioids, pleasant arousal with dopamine) and by hormones such as oestrogen and oxytocin (the so-called cuddle hormone).

The other instinctive systems are activated according to circumstances. PLAY: through rough and tumble play, all mammals practise social roles and conflict without risk. All the young romp around, which makes them happy.[37] As they mature, their play becomes more intricate and competitive. PLAY contributes to the emergence of complex communication and, thus, symbolic thinking.[38] The 'as if' nature of play suggests that PLAY may have been the biological precursor to thinking more broadly (i.e. to virtual rather than actual action).[39] Children love to play. Biologically, it involves testing boundaries of what is socially acceptable. Play often stops when such boundaries are crossed. It is also about exploring and establishing social relationships and hierarchies. Indeed, play often revolves around dominance and submission. This can be enjoyable to both parties as long as a certain balance is respected and each gets their share in terms of power. Taking the feelings of others into account is another evolutionary function of play. In humans, all this also takes shape within pretend play, where strength is tried out in different roles (e.g. Mother/Baby, Teacher/Pupil, Doctor/Patient, Cop/Robber, Cowboy/Indian). PLAY contributes to empathy. It is not an automatic phenomenon that can be attributed to mirror neurons, but it results from development and maturation.[40] In this context, I would like to refer to one of Winnicott's best-known statements. According to him, psychotherapy is essentially two people playing together.[41]

LUST makes mammals seek sexual partners, whereas pleasure shows the way to procreation. In LUST, there is a gender difference but male and female tendencies exist in both genders.[42] It is an emotional (and not a physical) instinct because you *can* survive without sex.[43] CARE is activated when we find a being in need. It plays a role in maternal love and the treatment of mainly pre-Oedipal patients who have missed something fundamental in this respect.[44] According to neuroscientist Patricia Churchland, it is difficult not to see this as a biological platform for morality.[45]

Mutatis mutandis, three pre-wired systems produce negative affects and thus prepare us for specific challenges. Threats mainly trigger FEAR, RAGE and PANIC/GRIEF. FEAR ensures that we are evolutionarily equipped to deal with dangers. It is the emotional drive that sets our minds to work. Instinctively, we freeze or run away when faced with danger to life or limb. Fear conditioning happens automatically without representation playing any role in it.[46] It does not involve the cortex. It is installed in the first years of life (Freud's period of infantile amnesia, which he attributed to the repression of the Oedipus complex) when the *hippocampus* (responsible for declarative memory) has not yet matured. Conditioning is virtually indelible; non-conscious memories are generally hard to forget. RAGE gives us the energy to fight threats, competition or injustice. It allows us to deter attackers when it is impossible to flee. It also allows us to rid ourselves of frustrating 'objects'. The famous *fight/flight* response refers to the combination of RAGE and FEAR, and the systems mentioned above are involved.[47]

Freud associates warfare with the death drive (which he came to understand as aggressive), but, for example, bearing in mind Jane Goodall's *Chimpanzee Wars*,[48] primates, too, being our closest relatives, battle over territory and social hierarchy. The higher the pecking order or, the higher the social status, the greater the ruler's rights to control the various resources available to the territory. As a hunter-gatherer, the male primate did not have to wait for an agricultural revolution to (want to) monopolise females either.

PANIC/GRIEF is triggered when we are abandoned. This system naturally underlies our vital need for attachment. It is complementary to CARE. There are distress vocalisations ('Mama!') upon separation so the youngster can be found again. Without a response, the youngster falls silent, according to Watt et al., to conserve energy and not wake sleeping dogs/predators.[49] After the Second World War, Darwin biographer John Bowlby extensively described this latter system with the response to separation and loss, going from protest to despair.[50] From a neuropsychoanalytic point of view, the drives of attachment and sexuality are distinct.[51] This has now been conclusively proven. In other words, authors such as Michael Balint, Ronald Fairbairn and the later object relation theorists were more than right.[52]

Johnson[53] uses the SEEKING system as an explanatory basis for libidinal cathexis. Within psychoanalysis, there are two fundamentally different assumptions: the subject is pleasure-seeking (drive theory), or it is object-seeking (object-relations theory). Today, the latter model takes precedence, and the drive has disappeared from the foreground.[54] However, the other six systems are indeed object-seeking or object-related. After all, their associated needs can only be met in the exterior world. Narcissistic or toxicogenic 'solutions' provide surrogate satisfaction but lead the subject down a *cul-de-sac* or side track. Note that this need not be attributed to the death drive but to the Ego employing wrong 'solutions'. The importance of the drive is consistent with the relational perspective. It only contributes to it and with some *sense of urgency* even. Much neurotic misery can be understood from the conflicting relationship between WANTING/SEEKING and LIKING.[55] The former pleasure has to do with appetite, the latter with consumption. The neurotic is typically feverishly seeking things that do not give him pleasure. Again drawing on Ariane Bazan, I will zoom in on this later.

Affect, Emotion and Feeling

In addition to the qualia or feeling qualities of affect,[56] biological needs acquire a hedonic valence so that increases or decreases in stress relative to deviation from homeostatic equilibria (or, looking ahead: increases or decreases in *prediction errors*) are felt as unpleasant and pleasant, respectively. In this, affective sensations like hunger and thirst differ from sensory sensations like seeing and hearing: seeing and hearing have no intrinsic value. Feelings do.[57] In Solms' view, the 'dawn of consciousness' involved little more than attributing hedonistic values to bodily sensations.[58] When philosopher and utilitarian Jeremy Bentham argued that 'nature had placed man under the governance of two masters: pleasure and pain', he was mistaken, for many animal brothers and sisters were already guided by these '*twin masters*' too.[59]

Each form of distress has a categorically different affective quality (hunger, thirst, fear, safety, sexuality and so on). Each set in motion species-specific programmes of action that are predicted to return the organism to more liveable limits. These behavioural programmes (intentional responses to sensory and emotional states) take the form of innate instincts and reflexes gradually elaborated and refined through experiential learning. This is Ego-development. The most important learning moments occur during critical periods, such as early childhood, when we cannot deal with often clashing emotional instincts or affects. We must compromise and invent or discover indirect or symbolic-imaginary ways to satisfy our needs and desires. The fact that our phenomenal consciousness senses fluctuations in its own needs allows choices to be made in all respects. It is helpful for survival and procreation in an environment or context that was not predicted. Behold, according to Solms, the biological why of subjective experience and perception once again.

Emotion is a sense that registers not the external but the internal world. How *are* you? The heart of the matter is expressed very well in French: *Comment ça va?*[60] How's (your) Id? While external events may trigger emotions, they reflect your feelings. This is expressed in our facial expressions or motor skills and is perceptible to others, so (thanks to mirror neurons, among other things) empathic responses can (but will not always) occur. But internal (vaso-)motor changes may not be registered and translated centrally.

For those to whom this all sounds rather primitive: is our emotional life so simple? By no means. Nelleke Nicolai,[61] for example, makes a further distinction between affects, emotions and feelings. Affects are unconscious reactions to internal stimuli. They manifest physically through palpitations, perspiring, redness, buckling knees, an urge to defecate, etc. Affects, in a sense, are pre-personal. They are the body's way of preparing for evolutionarily necessary action. Emotions are partly unconscious but also already partially conscious responses to stimuli. They also have more or less social content. Only feelings are emotions to which a particular meaning can be assigned. They are personal and situated in a historical-biographical context. Through inner sensation (called interoception), you can discover how good or bad you feel, but to know *what* you think (exactly) and thus to read your own emotions requires intersubjective experience from infancy onwards. This emotional literacy occurs only in joint (ad-)ventures with others.[62] Awareness, distinguishing from consciousness, and subjective signification of affects and emotions depend on development and life/learning history.[63]

Primary emotions serve procreation or survival. Subcortical areas drive them. They are made more complex by the alloys they form with each other or secondary or tertiary elaboration. For example, fear and anger are primary feelings and guilt and shame are secondary feelings: alloys of primary or hybrid emotions in which specific cognitions also come into play.[64] Conditioning and other rudimentary forms of emotional learning leave their mark on them. The *amygdala* and *hippocampus*, in particular, fulfil a leading role. Tertiary emotions are cognitively 'bound' feelings and thoughts, primarily controlled cortically by the medial-frontal cortex and the limbic system. The frontal lobe regulates but does not generate emotions. Some emotions do have a *very* pronounced and sophisticated neocortical aspect. I will give just two examples for which John Koenig[65] came up with numerous amusing neologisms. For instance, there is *ellipsis*: a word that describes the sad feeling that can be triggered by knowing you won't be able to experience certain things in the future. Or *liberosis*: the wish many people have when they long to be children again and not have to care about anything anymore. It is occasionally enough to read a novel by Gustave Flaubert or Jonathan Franzen to enjoy the emotional panoply and the kaleidoscopic light thrown on people's emotional lives. Of course, listening to what people freely associate can also be helpful for this purpose.

So, with permission, I will go a little further. Qualia are negative if they deviate from a homeostatic equilibrium (and thus -as we will see shortly- increase entropy/uncertainty), and the opposite is true for positive qualia. There are many flavours of qualia, each expressing its individual need and allowing the organism to make judgements with minimal computational effort.[66] All needs cannot be felt at the same time; much less alleviated. Priorities must be set according to the specific context (balancing of needs and needs versus opportunities). Emotions must therefore be expanded through external perception or exteroception: they must be contextualised:[67] I feel this way about this and that way about that. In other words, they must be processed by cognitive consciousness and 'bound' by it. This corresponds precisely to what Freud called the secondary process in 1915, which, after all, involves the 'binding' of the primary form of drive energy, which can move freely: 'I believe that this distinction [between bound and free energy] is so far our deepest insight into the nature of nervous energy, and I do not see how it could be ignored'.[68]

Biology: Homeostasis

From Jaak Panksepp and Antonio Damasio, Solms had already concluded that sub-jective feelings must somehow result from homeostatic processes. Such homeo-static equilibria also operate in emotional affects. They do not relate to bodily but to object-relational 'needs'. We also have 'expected states' regarding attachment, care, sexuality or play, and deviation from these makes themselves felt. This even-tually led Solms to realise that Freud's definition of the drive as the 'measure of the demand made upon the mind for work '[69] corresponds to so-called *error* signals. Thus, he ended up with Freud's insights from his *Project*. He considered bodily needs to be the driving forces of our mental life and the forebrain merely a sym-pathetic ganglion that monitors and regulates the drive. Homeostatic equilibrium points are nothing other than the *expected states* of the organism. Homeostasis keeps the organism within certain limits. RAGE is about ensuring that nothing should stand in my way, FEAR that nothing threatens my survival or bodily pre-servation. Moreover, unlike the thermostat in our living room, our lives depend on it. When abnormal, there are error signals that either trigger autonomous regulation (e.g. to regulate blood pressure) or -certainly in the case of emotional instincts-reach consciousness when real work is to be done. Solms prefers to speak of needs in the former (autonomous) case; in the latter (mental) case, he likes to talk of drives. The distinction rests mainly in the degree of uncertainty. Regulating blood pressure is much simpler than ensuring you get a partner willing to have sex with you, conceive children and take care of them with you. All drives are homeostatic, but the emotional ones do not have physical but object-relational origins. It is much more difficult and complex to satisfy them. They constantly and inevitably collide, especially in our love and relational life (care, grief, sex, play, seeking and so on).[70]

Feelings enable more complex organisms to register deviation from homeo-static equilibria in non-predicted environments, thus regulating and prioritising behaviour through thought and random action. These organisms can learn from experience thanks to this. In predictable conditions, they can return to reflexive or automated responses (also selected by natural selection). In novel situations, however, the organism must be able to orient itself in the here and now based on value judgements according to valence, and so-called free will plays a (more prominent) role.[71] In all this, the organism has to stay ahead of the wave of bio-logically pre-programmed (re-)action programmes and 'surf on uncertainty', so to speak, as Andy Clark aptly put it in 2016.[72]

To Solms, following Damasio, consciousness is a way of monitoring our internal state. The brainstem does this silently: organising temperature, glucose, salt, water, and so on is regulated automatically/by the autonomic nervous system (the physiological unconscious). All this becomes conscious only when action needs to be taken. In his many lectures on *YouTube,* Solms gives the example of a building on fire. Sooner or later, you will smell danger and spring into action. You navigate the building using your shortness of breath and sensitivity to heat as a compass to save your skin *along the way*. This is drive and homeostasis in their standard form. Our ideal is that everything comes naturally/is fully automated. (How is Id? Ça va!). Freud's constancy or even Nirvana principle applies more specifically to an Ego that navigates life effortlessly. Solms refers to a song by *Talking Heads*, when he compares it to a heaven, where nothing ever happens.[73] This is because everything is 'settled' there thanks to automated (autonomous or automatable) predictions. When we are banned from (this) 'heaven', I might refer to James Joyce, who puts it a bit dramatically: 'First, we feel, then we fall'.[74]

Conversely, SEEKING is the result of free energy prompting activity. We are unhappy and dissatisfied because we need something even though we don't realise precisely what we need. The other emotional systems drive SEEKING. However, note that the outcome is not always happy because we can become fixated on 'bad' solutions due to adverse experiences in our history and its object relations. If we find ourselves somehow *between a rock and a hard place*, we may 'choose' (with all its adverse consequences) and become fixated on the proverbial One-Eyed King (or Queen) in the Land of the Blind. The monstrosity of this cyclops is then sometimes lost sight of. We cling to 'wrong' solutions or 'bad' objects simply because they gave us some adaptive advantage at one time (and in the circumstances given at the time).

The fact that it is good to survive and procreate implies a biologically based value system by which positive feelings are linked to certain adaptive behaviours. This does not mean that we have sex to serve our biological interests. We have sex simply because we find it pleasurable and not because of evolutionary interests. The arousal we experience is a predictor of gratification. Still, the latter implies the little death (French: *la petite mort* as a term for orgasm) of gratification and serves the Nirvana principle. This brings us back to the so-called death drive, which, in a sense, helps the life drive. Life leads to death, but it does not strive for death. It seeks only (and even with excitement) discharge/gratification.[75] Both are very much worth repeating. After all, as Friedrich Nietzsche noted: *Alle Lust will Ewigkeit, will tiefe, tiefe Ewigkeit.*[76] All pleasure wants eternity, wants deep, deep eternity.

Endnotes

1 Evolutionary theory (like psychoanalysis) has now been extensively labelled and clarified (see, for instance, Jablonka and Lamb (2005)) but its main premises remain intact. The overly neo-Darwinian emphasis on genes is in need of revision. Geneticists named isolate four modes of inheritance: genetic, epigenetic (*nurture* influences), behavioural and symbolic variation.

2 Darwin (1981 [1871], p. 85). Pointing briefly to a fundamentalist opposite (Žižek 1997, p. 32) for whom the Lacanian subject of the unconscious means not the pre-discursive reservoir of affects and drives but the exact opposite: a purely logical construction. Marc De Kesel (2009) introduces the Munchhausen paradigm in this context: the subject pulling itself out of the swamp by its own hair/signifiers.

3 Darwin (1981 [1871], p. 488).

4 Freud (1940a, p. 449, 1940b, p. 147)

5 Darwin *The Origin of Species* (facsimile edition first edition) pp. 22–23).

6 His *The Hidden Spring* is even dedicated to Jaak Panksepp.

7 Panksepp (2007).

8 Panksepp and Biven (2012, p. 25).

9 Panksepp (2011). See also Nicolai (2014, p. 282) for a diagram of this *nested brain hierarchy*.

10 Kinet (2021a).

11 Skinner (2005 [1953]).

12 Within psychotherapy, it is important to maintain a fundamental distinction between feelings and behaviour. We have no voluntary control over feelings. There is no button to turn them on/off nor to regulate their volume. In general, they do get tempered to the extent that we can access them (better) with our reason. In a one-liner, psychotherapy is using your reason to understand your feelings. On the other hand, we are and remain responsible for our behaviour, except in cases of insanity. Even if our behaviour is 'unintentional'.

13 Thorndike (1911).

14 Solms (2021d, p. 108).

15 Ibid., p. 122.

16 Sitskoorn (2006, 2010).

17 Rudimentary sketches on brain anatomy can easily be found on the Internet. For this, see also Panksepp (1998), and Damasio (2010).

18 Solms (2013a).

19 Dawkins (1996).

20 This terminology is explained later.

21 Kandel (2012). All psychopharmaceuticals act in this zone.

22 Jane Goodall and Frans De Waal are considered the most prominent primatologists. I referred to the relevance of this science in Kinet (2019). Genetically, the difference between homo sapiens and primates is as small or large as that between the African and the Indian elephant.

23 De Waal (2017).

24 Krupenye et al. (2016).

25 Peña-Guzmán (2022).

26 Andrews-Hanna et al. (2010)

27 Buckner, Andrews-Hanna and Schacter (2008).

28 Ekman (2013).

29 Eagle (2011, p. 252).

30 Solms (2021e, p. 1071).

31 Panksepp (1998, p. 144) and see also Yu (2001b), Solms (2018b). Libido, on the other hand, is related to Lacanian *jouissance*.

32 Panksepp (1971).

33 Solms (2021e, p. 1068).

34 Solms and Turnbull (2002), Solms and Zellner (2012a).

35 When discussing Lacanian *jouissance*, I will henceforth use the somewhat archaic term 'enjoyment'. *Jouissance* can initially be defined pragmatically as the unconscious benefit that specific behaviour provides so that it persists even when it is no longer 'healthy' (or even harmful/lethal) (Evans 1996, p. 92; Lacan 1986, p. 209).

36 Burgdorf and Panksepp (2006), Siviy and Panksepp (2011).
37 Revelling is the 'rough and tumble play' we have in common with most mammals, and that helps us experiment with social roles, power relations, rules of play, sublimation and symbolism and so on.
38 I refer to the famous statement by German Romantic philosopher Friedrich Schiller ([2016] 1794) in his *On the Aesthetic Education of Man*: 'Man is never so authentically himself than when at play'.
39 Solms (2021d, p. 145).
40 Solms (2017a).
41 Winnicott (1971).
42 Solms (2018b, 2018c).
43 Solms (2021e, p. 1065).
44 Balint (1968).
45 Churchland (2022, p. 44): 'The mother defends the baby, stays with the baby even when the baby is a great bloody nuisance. The mother takes risks for the baby and sacrifices her own interests for the baby; we know human mothers and fathers do that all the time. The idea really is that when you see what the neurochemistry does in terms of what we call attachment, but what really translates into this kind of caring and cooperating behaviour, it is hard not to see that as a platform for morality'.
46 LeDoux (1996).
47 Panksepp and Biven (2012, p. 200).
48 Goodall (1986).
49 Watt and Panksepp (2009).
50 'Grief is shut-down SEEKING, and full-blast SEEKING is mania before it tips into psychosis' Solms (2021e, p. 1075).
51 Bowlby (1969, 1973).
52 Solms (2021e, p. 1076).
53 Johnson (2008). We wish the other *bon appétit* and not *bon faim*, because the meal revolves around enjoyment rather than satisfaction (of a need).
54 Eagle (2011, p. 54).
55 Robinson and Berridge (1993).
56 Thomas Nagel (2012) mainly introduced the 'qualia'. They include, for example, the experience of pain, drinking a glass of wine or listening to Bach.
57 Solms (2021d, p. 117).
58 Ibid., p. 124.
59 Robinson (1973, p. 119).
60 Le Ça as das Es, the Id.
61 Nicolai (2017).
62 I explained this in more detail in Kinet (2010c). Allan Schore (1994, 2003a, 2003b), in particular, researched the neurobiology of attachment. Psychoanalytic theory and mother-child observations are then combined with functional MRI. The early social environment of so-called *primary caretakers* turns out to have a direct influence on the brain structures responsible for socio-emotional development. Right hemispheric communication between the mother and (only her!) baby, in particular, plays a key role in this (especially in the first eighteen-thirty-six months of life).
63 Tsakiris and Critchley (2016). Let me give a simple example. A person can behave nervously without being aware of this nervousness: affect. That same person can feel nervous: emotion. Finally, that same person can give meaning to his nervousness: I am anxious, irritated, miffed, excited and so on.
64 Solms (2021d, p. 139).
65 Koenig (2022).

66 Solms and Friston (2018, note 7).
67 One of the ills of an overly medically inspired mental health service: the de-contextualisation of problems.
68 Freud (1915c, p. 87, 1915d, p. 187).
69 Freud (1915a, 1915b).
70 Solms (2021e, p. 1062).
71 Solms (2013).
72 Clark (2016).
73 Joyce (2020 [1939]).
74 Solms (2019a, note 45).
75 Solms (2021e, pp. 1053–1054).
76 Nietzsche (2022 [1885]) in *Also sprach Zarathustra*.

Chapter 10

Interlude

Infinitely Less Than Zero

There are two pillars in psychoanalysis. The clinical describes empirically observable phenomena and processes, whereas the metapsychological postulates (more or less speculatively) the working laws behind them. One is close to experience, the other distant from it. Some psychoanalysts prefer to dwell in the former, others in the latter domain. Ideally, the two should go together. After all, we can only help people properly if we can also grasp the fundamental workings of their minds. This requires not only an ideographic but also a nomothetic approach. Paraphrasing Marx, there is nothing more practical than a good theory.

As psychoanalysts, we are all well-versed in primary and secondary process thinking. The primary process is that which dominates our dream life, that is, our unconscious. In a free-energy flux and an associative chain, condensation and displacement play a crucial role. The pleasure principle is a thermostat in this process. Living beings are negentropic and, in terms of tension, strive not for zero but constancy. The secondary process is that of conscious thought: linguistic and rational, answering to Aristotelian logic. Here, the pleasure principle remains operative, but it is lifted to the reality principle, which is an extension of it.

In his metapsychological text on the unconscious, Freud further distinguishes between unconscious, pre-conscious and conscious. The pre-conscious can be recalled. The unconscious is separated from it by a barrier of repression. Most dreams we cannot remember. We can try to hold on to them, but because of some weird memory disorder, they often slip through our fingers irrevocably – against our will. They are volatile.

In his text on repression, Freud distinguishes between primal repression and the actual postrepression. In the first case, contents have not been conscious (linguistically) at any time. They do not enter the narrative, but their representation and charge persist unchanged and continue to leave their decisive mark. In present terms, this memory is not explicit but implicit. It is non-declarative. You can neither tell nor retell it. It emerges only under the guise of (repeated) action.

The second repression stage involves thought processes associatively intertwined with the primal repressed. Therefore, they undergo the same fate as the primal repressed. While primal repression is about not being able to know, repression is about not wanting or not being allowed to know. The repression referred to

DOI: 10.4324/9781003394358-10

when it comes to defence mechanisms is a postrepression. It can be assisted and supported by other defence mechanisms, such as projection, reaction formation, rationalisation or intellectualisation.

After Freud, the unconscious was given many other interpretations such as, for example, the cognitive (descriptive) unconscious, the physiological (of our auto-nomic nervous system and vegetative processes), the ideological (the implicit cul-ture that quasi-naturally determines our comings and goings) or that of attachment (which is passed down through generations like a counting-out). Each of them determines our life, albeit without our knowledge.

Even with Freud, the unconscious already had a variety of meanings: descrip-tive, dynamic and systemic. In his structural model, Id, Ego and Superego appear to have unconscious, pre-conscious and conscious aspects. The Id is not the linguistic law-driven domain of the dream but a pool of seething urges bubbling up from our bodies into the unconscious.

The same amount of conceptual confusion developed over time between me, the Ego, the Self and the subject, and the overlap between the Id and the uncon-scious consequently became a foggy domain. Is the unconscious internal, or does it reside in a field/zone around/between us? Jacques Lacan indicates that inside and outside blend with his neologism of *extimacy* or his image of the Möbius band.[1] To him, primordial *extimacy* is same-born with our entry into (symbolic) language which, after all, does not record everything in its register. It is the real that never wholly (as opposed to entirely never) gets bound to symbolic-imaginary repre-sentations. For Bion, too, not all experience is 'alphabetised'. What he calls beta elements persist (in the absence of alpha function or reverie of the big Other) in us and unconsciously exert their disruptive effects.

Two contemporary psychoanalysts use a model completing both of these per-spectives. The Canadian Joseph Fernando introduces the concept of zero-process concerning trauma.[2] The Flemish Bion expert Rudi Vermote speaks of an undiffer-entiated zone of infinity in our psyche.[3] For him, empirical neuroscience replaces metapsychology. He does not refer to trauma but to the domain of psychosis and the pre-verbal. It is the primordial oceanic soup in which molecules have conglo-merated into primitive life forms.

In Freud's *The Interpretation of Dreams*, there already was a fledgling idea of a symbolising function of the dream that precedes the pleasure principle. After Freud, the focus shifted towards the ability to dream rather than decoding the dream. If beta elements do not get 'dreamed', they continue to assail us mutely and disturbingly. Freud's rejection and evacuating forms of projective identification (as opposed to symbolisation) are the rules. Fernando here refers to zero-process thinking. The raw and traumatic experience is repeated (not similarly but identi-cally). This repetition compulsion can be broken only through the salutary inter-vention of the reverie/alpha function.

Most psychoanalysts equate deep, early and severe psychopathological pheno-mena. According to Fernando, however, even later, trauma can catapult us back to the psychological stone age. The contents of the zero-process remain in a frozen state.

They lack the continuous movement and interaction characteristic of the displacements and condensations of the primary process. They also need the secondary process's higher integrations, abstractions and linguistic thinking. Zero-processes are the domain of the fatally diabolic (etymologically: what separates/splits).

The model proposed by Rudi Vermote also involves a psychic functioning in different layers: from undifferentiated/infinite to differentiated/finite. Starting from Freud's structural model of the psyche, Vermote arrives at a threefold division: the conscious, the repressed and the primal unconscious. The last is the unknowable unconscious, where there is no representation yet, with formless and undifferentiated emotional experiences.

Following Matte-Blanco and Bion, Vermote finds the gradient infinite–finite more valuable than the unconscious–conscious distinction. The finite layers represent reason and logical thinking. The intermediate zone (with mixed finite and infinite layers) represents dreams, free association and play, and the infinite represents feelings, experiences and intuition. The infinite lack causal connections, for example, because 'part of the infinite is also infinite'. On the other hand, the conscious, linguistic and secondary process can be compared to the finite because it does have fixed connections.

To Fernando, the petrification of trauma must be 'liquified' by the psychoanalytic couple's saliva and other digestive juices. To Vermote, both parties of the psychoanalytic couple must seek the (sometimes terrifying) frontier of the infinite to allow new and more fruitful bonds and connections to emerge.

We can speculatively contrast Fernando and Vermote as follows. Fernando's zero-process is characterised by petrification and repetition, while in Vermote's concept, infinite fluidity and dissolution predominate. The primary process is dominated by association, and binding is at its zenith. In the secondary process, argumentation and connection are the rules. Driving through all this is a gradient from high to low entropy and, in Freud's terminology, from death drive to life drive.

Allegedly, you have to make things as simple as possible but not simpler. Generating a maximum of meaning with a minimum of signifiers also provides (economic) pleasure. This text oscillates deliberately between pleasure and reality, seduction and education. It '*seducates*' between two chairs and beside the psychoanalytic couch.[4]

Endnotes

1 If we glue the ends of a strip of paper together, the result is a ring with one inside and one outside. If, before glueing the ends together, we first turn one of the ends one turn, a so-called Möbius band is created. As the inside and outside now merge, only one side remains. If you slide your finger along this ring, you go unnoticed on the other side. This movement makes tangible how relative opposites can be.

2 Fernando (2018).

3 Vermote (2015).

4 Beside the Couch (*Naast de bank*) is a regular section of the Dutch *Journal of Psychoanalysis* (*Tijdschrift voor Psychoanalyse*): short texts on psychoanalytic asides.

Chapter 11

To Consciousness

In Search of the Soul

Now that I have explained in detail why the drive is rising again, we ascend to Solms' findings and views on consciousness. If we first unpack 'consciousness' as a concept, it has several meanings. Consciousness in its first meaning (consciousness as a waking state) is a necessary condition for consciousness in its second meaning: consciousness as experience, also called phenomenal consciousness. The latter, in turn, must be distinguished from secondary or 'reflective' consciousness (knowing that and what you are hearing, seeing, feeling or thinking). This secondary consciousness is the pain that separates us from ourselves. It is mainly in this latter sense that to be conscious/aware of something is used by psychoanalysis. It largely coincides with that which we can put into words. That's why I often refer to a saying by Dada poet Tristan Tzara in one of his Manifestoes: '*La pensée se fait dans la* bouche'.[1] Thought is formed (I would add: only) in the mouth (or pen, of course).

Because intelligence is located in the cortex and occupies such a large volume in human brains, it was assumed that our consciousness was located there for a long time. But we now know that consciousness is much more primitive and that we have had it in common with vertebrates for hundreds of millions of years. It tells you how you are, and it helps you make sure you are well. According to affective scientists such as Antonio Damasio, Jaak Panksepp and Björn Merker, consciousness in its elementary form is feeling.[2] Like Freud, they place the importance of feelings above that of cognition. English philosopher David Hume was right back in 1739: 'Reason is, and ought only to be, the slave of the passions'.[3]

During the past decades, there has been a frantic search for the *neural correlate of consciousness* (NCC). In 1994, DNA discoverer Francis Crick called it *The Scientific Search for the Soul*. Cognitive science based its search on visual information processing, which has, after all, been mapped in more detail than any other modality of consciousness. Meanwhile, however, our smartphone also recognises our fingerprints or faces. This information is processed in the dark, without inner feeling. Therefore, the analogy with the computer is a poor metaphor for the relationship between brain and mind.

DOI: 10.4324/9781003394358-11

Philosopher David Chalmers[4] regards the search for the neural correlate of our consciousness as the 'easy' problem. After all, its discovery would (only) explain where and not how or why consciousness arises. Current computer technology has developed language, memory and perception. It can discriminate, categorise and respond to environmental stimuli, but none of this is sufficient to assume that it *feels* like something for the computer to speak, remember or perceive. For Chalmers, this is the 'hard problem': how and why do neurophysiological activities produce such a thing as conscious experience? Philosopher Thomas Nagel had also asked himself this question long before. I quote: 'As far as I can imagine (and very far it is not), I only come to know what it would be like for *me* to behave like a bat. But that is not the question. I want to know what it is like *for a bat* to be a bat'.[5] An organism has conscious mental states only if the sensation of being itself exists. In other words, the hard problem concerns the subjective experiences that spring from objective neurophysiological processes. Although these experiences (qualia or phenomenal consciousness) presumably have a physical basis – there is no consciousness without a brain – the question of how and why remains. A thought experiment known as the Knowledge Argument may reveal how critical consciousness is.[6] A blind neuroscientist named Mary knows everything about the eye, light, colours, the visual cortex, etc. Only when she can see at a certain point does she discover a whole new body of knowledge that she had been missing until then: how it *feels* when you see the colour red.

On the other hand, one of the most important lessons of cognitive science is that cognitions (perception, learning, memory and so on) typically occur (descriptively) unconsciously. There is constant 'perception without awareness of what is perceived, learning without awareness of what is learned'.[7] At most, five per cent of our psychological functioning is conscious, and cognitions become aware only to the extent we need them to be. A review article in *American Psychologist,* with a nod to Milan Kundera, thus mentions '*The unbearable automaticity of being*'.[8]

Cognition, perception, thinking, remembering or judging can all occur unconsciously/in the dark. It is only when the brain stem activates the cortex that the screen flashes on and the film (Wilfred Bion: of waking dream thought)[9] constantly playing in the background becomes visible. The feeling also sets the tone of this screen. I will skip from the neural to the clinical situation for a moment. Every psychotherapy session is couched in a particular emotional tone. Tuning into the correct wavelength is essential for proper understanding. Solms explains well that two distinct neural processes interact here: fast synaptic transmission (from on/off switches) and slower waves of (affective) postsynaptic neuromodulation that are gradual, emanate from our bodies (pituitary, adrenal, thyroid, gonads and *hypothalamus*) and determine the affective keynote by influencing the likelihood of a particular group of neurons being activated.[10] They decide in which key the notes/needs are set ... and must be understood.

Evolutionarily, we must view consciousness archaeologically as consisting of different layers or sediments. Most fundamental are the urges that drive us and other animals to go out into the outside world to tap all kinds of resources. Hunger, lust or fear drive us to restore homeostasis. In fear, we empty our bowels, and a surge of neuronal activity in our *amygdala* and *hypothalamus* makes us flee or freeze. A feedback loop develops between these older responses and a higher level in mammals. Fear, for example, becomes more specific (rats are afraid of light and humans of the dark): the same fear system kicks in but in response to different 'threats'. A third layer superimposes itself on this in humans, namely between rational/cognitive processes and lower-level triggers and learned mechanisms. Fear then becomes intertwined with conceptual and narrative thinking. Speech, symbols and language, increased skills, mastery and future planning may draw on emotions and energies of lower layers, but these achieve a typically human sophistication.

Antonio Damasio[11] had already developed a theory of our consciousness as consisting of three chronological and hierarchical layers: proto-self, core consciousness and extended consciousness. The proto-self is a coherent neural pattern continuously monitoring the organism's physical structure. For this, neuroanatomically necessary and homologous structures throughout the species are the *hypothalamus* (which manages the organism's homeostasis), the brainstem (the nuclei which pick up body signals) and the insular cortex, which connects all this with emotions. This is followed by the core consciousness that emerges when the organism becomes aware of feelings related to its inner bodily state. It experiences thoughts as its own and develops an ephemeral sense of self, using the continuous production of representations based on information from the proto-self. Thus, this level of consciousness is not the privilege of man. It remains stable throughout the organism's lifetime. Only when consciousness expands beyond the here and now does Damasio's third and final layer of consciousness emerge: the *extended consciousness* that occurs only in humans.

Mark Es

In line with his contemporaries, Freud had equated conscious and Ego on the one hand and unconscious and Id on the other. He tied in with the localising brain anatomy that situated the seat of consciousness in the cerebral cortex, in the outer, enveloping layer of the central organ. Still, according to Freud, conscious feelings, like perceptions, emanated from the Ego (the part of the mind he situated in the cerebral cortex), not from the unconscious Id, which had to be located in the brain stem and *hypothalamus*. In short: Freud had misplaced the functional relationship between the Id (the brain stem) and the Ego (the cerebral cortex), at least where feelings were concerned. He thought the perceiving Ego was conscious and the feeling Id was unconscious.[12]

In his seminal article '*The Conscious Id*', Mark Solms explains how he calls the Id *conscious*, completely contradicting Freud. To do so, he again employs Teuber's evidence of double dissociation.[13] The affect is thereby re-located according to the reasoning that function A is lost due to damage to structure X but not structure Y, and function B is lost due to damage to structure Y but not structure X (with A = consciousness, B = cognition, X = brainstem and Y = cortex). Decorticated cats appear to be as lively as cats with cortices.[14] Babies born with hydranencephaly (i.e. without cortex) respond affectively adequately to stimuli and environmental factors.[15] Solms presents several case studies, e.g. a patient with massive cortical cerebral infarction who responds pertinently and even wittily to all questions (probing for subjectivity and awareness).[16]

Conversely, in humans and vertebrates, not the cortex but the ERTAS (extended reticular–thalamic activating system or RAS for short) appears to be the neuronal correlate for consciousness. This reticular formation is found in all vertebrates, from fish to humans, and must therefore be around 525 million years old.[17] A lesion in this subcortical structure produces immediate coma. Still, this is not just an on/off switch. For this reason, this ERTAS is not only relevant to anaesthetists but also to psychiatrists. All drugs that act on the neurotransmitters located in the brain nuclei of the ERTAS (such as serotonin, dopamine, noradrenaline or acetylcholine) have substantial effects on anxiety and mood, which is why they make up the lion's share of psychiatric pharmacotherapy. With dorsal electrical stimulation of the (subcortical) periaqueductal grey, immediate melancholic depression with suicidal tendencies occurs, and with ventral stimulation, immediate feelings of euphoria and bliss.

Consciousness is affective. Full stop. From studies of lesions, deep brain stimulation, pharmacological agents and functional imaging studies, one conclusion forces itself upon us. In the reticular nucleus of the brain stem, not only consciousness arises but also affect.[18] All affective circuits converge in this one structure (as big as the head of a match): the periaqueductal grey (PAG), the leading centre for producing feelings and emotion-driven behaviour. It is not strictly part of the RAS, although it is directly adjacent and closely linked to it.[19] Although the PAG is anatomically subcortical, it is at the top functionally. According to Björn Merker, it forms the affective-sensory-motor pivot or interface of the brain's 'decision triangle'.[20] And to Panksepp, this primal self is the ultimate source of our subjective, sentient being.[21] The error signals from our physical and emotional needs enter the PAG. This ancient core of the brain stem continuously receives information from the outside world (current opportunities) and from the inside world (current needs), and efferent pathways also depart in the direction of the locomotor centres. Thus, it is a platform where a choice is made among the various error signals fired from the different homeostatic interests. Priorities have to be set (food or sex, sleep or flight), and this is done based on salience. What maximises reduction in free energy or surprise? What is prioritised manifests as a drive that determines our voluntary behaviour at that moment, while all other interests are automatically or autonomously pursued.[22]

According to Solms, the subcortical circuits do the same intellectual work as the Id.[23] They evolved this way to ensure the individual's well-being and promote procreation. As Freud[24] described it, the Id is filled with energy derived from drives but not organised. The pleasure principle rules; it operates only in the here and now, and there is only striving for immediate satisfaction. There are no logical laws, and in particular, no contradiction. Various drive claims exist side by side without erasing or diminishing each other. At most, they may converge into an alloy, a composite or a 'compromise' according to the quantitatively/economically dominant 'partial drive'.[25]

The Id is the needy/desiring part of the mind. Survival/self-preservation and procreation/sexuality are the predominant motifs there. Roughly speaking, it is located in the brainstem, *hypothalamus*, ventral *striatum* and *amygdala*. Meanwhile, according to the 2012 *Cambridge Declaration on Consciousness*, there is consensus within the global scientific community that 'the *absence of a neocortex does not appear to preclude an organism from experiencing affective states*'.[26] Stephen Hawking also endorsed this text, but animal rights' implications have barely hit home...

And I

The capacities of the neocortex (reality testing, planning, mastery, impulse control) can all be reduced to the so-called Ego functions.[27] According to Freud, the Ego is part of the Id that changes due to contact with the outside world. It receives and protects against stimuli and develops representations on behalf of the Id that would otherwise constantly and blindly bump into reality (like an ant against an obstacle).

In a famous statement, the Ego is, to Freud, first and foremost, a body-Ego. It is not so much a superficial entity as the projection of a (bodily) surface.[28] Self and object representations are cortical. They stabilise our experiences. Energy is bound there, and the future (of our object relations, too)[29] is made predictable. Registration of exteroceptive experiences also takes place cortically, namely by this (body) Ego. Thinking/cognition can be repressed, and feelings are decapitated by it but continue to wander, orphaned, through the psyche in search of (so to speak) hooks to hang from. Lifting repression means reassigning our feelings to the 'right' places (again).

The Ego is executive and regulatory. It maps the outside world and mediates impulses coming from the Id. To this end, it can control, learn and predict. It can operate according to the reality principle thanks to a space it creates between drive claims and (motor or other) action. This Ego is embodied by the primary sensory-motor and virtually the whole neocortex. The Superego grafts itself onto the Ego with commandments and prohibitions. It results from identifications with or internalisations of social rules, not least on account of parents. Neuroanatomically, it sits on the oldest portions of the association cortex, the brainstem and *basal ganglia*, where functional integration occurs.

Consciousness comes from exteroception, but consciousness is endogenous and merely causes the activation/awareness of cortical representations. In this, we should always remember that cortical perception is always *apperception*. What appears in consciousness, after all, are not direct, unprocessed signals from the periphery but predictive inferences from the memory traces of those signals and their consequences. Our perceptions of the here and now are guided by predictions derived mainly from long-term memory.[30]

Memories, therefore, are not simply data from the past. Biologically, they are about the past, but they serve the future. Every memory is a prediction meant to meet our needs. To save energy, the brain sends in only that part of the incoming information that does *not* match expectations. Stable cortical inferences are provided with sensation, creating fixed mental representations of the external world as it manifests in our heads. Solms calls them 'mental solids'[31] The feeling is only bound and stabilised by cortico-thalamic processing. The affect was raw and unbound. The so-called level of consciousness is due to varying free energy. In thermodynamic terms, this is called entropy, and in information-theoretic terms, it involves surprise (or uncertainty), which is expressed neurophysiologically as *arousal*.[32]

Since we never manage to make completely flawless predictions, SEEKING is the predominant/'default' drive: a positive relationship to uncertainty to address it proactively. When this affect predominates, it feels like curiosity and interest in what is going on in the world. You may then be called a 'seeker' by those around you.

Drives and their associated affects are the causal mechanisms of consciousness, both in its physiological and psychological guise. The underlying mechanisms might be reducible to physical laws, as described by Karl Friston. They underlie self-organisation. Consciousness is not something above or beyond nature, but it is part of nature, and the book of nature is written (paraphrasing Galileo Galilei) in the language of mathematics.

Physics: Entropy

The connecting factor between the biological approach of affective neuroscience and Karl Friston's physics input is homeostasis.[33] The entirely new inspirations the latter brought are entropy and its information-theoretic *counterpart*, namely surprise or uncertainty. After all, in the latter capacity, entropy refers not only to the physical material but also to virtual or mental phenomena or contents of consciousness.

Entropy is a concept from physics and, more specifically, thermodynamics. Its first law is that of conservation of energy. No energy can be added; nothing arises from nothing. Nor can energy be destroyed. One form of energy can be transformed into another state, but according to the second law, in the process, a part is permanently transformed into a form that can no longer be used. Physical processes are always irreversible, and energy constantly changes from a 'useable' to a 'less useable' form. It does not disappear, nor is it destroyed – see the first law – but changes into a state where labour can no longer be supplied. This unusable energy is called entropy. In the universe, this entropy or disorder is constantly increasing. Its ultimate consequence will be the so-called heat death, in which nothing more can happen because no more labour can be supplied.

We could also think of entropy as the number of places each atom or molecule can be at a given time. In thermodynamics, we speak of Helmholtz free energy; in chemistry of Gibbs free energy and in information theory, we talk about Friston free energy.[34] This takes us into the realm of probability theory. This is important because, unlike the other laws of thermodynamics, the laws of probability apply to everything, not just material things. Not only can the entropy of a room filled with gas be defined in terms of probability, but the same can also be done with the entropy of a psychological decision-making process. In both cases, the entropy increases with the increased randomness of the possible outcomes. The 'entropy' of the dispersing gas cloud is the same entropy as that of the expansion of the number of possible options. Not everything in nature is visible or tangible, but everything is subject to the laws of probability. This is why probability theory goes to the heart of modern physics, in which matter is no longer a basic concept and from which classical particles have disappeared.[35]

That feeling signals homeostatic anomalies and prediction errors became clear to Solms only after he delved into the work of Karl Friston, starting in 2010. At first, Friston's publications were inscrutable, but Solms grasped the essence, especially after reading a 2013 article entitled '*Life as we know it*'.[36] In this article, Friston tries to capture nothing less than the difference between living and non-living things in mathematical equations. It revolves around the laws that drive homeostasis: the tendency of living things to resist entropy and maintain equilibria in multiple ways and changing conditions.

According to Friston, the fundamental driving force of all life forms is that they are obliged to minimise their free energy. This obligation determines all their actions. It is a homeostatic (cf Freud's constancy) principle, but it goes further than that. Friston explains that biological systems (like cells) must have arisen through complicated variants of the process by which simpler 'self-organising' systems arose (like crystals from liquid). According to him, the same mechanism is involved, namely the 'minimisation of free energy', which I will return to in a moment. All self-organising systems (ourselves included) have one all-important task in common: to persist.

It also explains the self-organisation[37] by which proto-life formed from the primordial soup. It is the way a self forms, namely through the formation of what is called a Markov blanket. I got stuck with this strange blanket in Solms' *The Hidden Spring*. I compare it, metaphorically and in simplified form, to what distinguishes a cloud (according to physical laws) from the surrounding non-cloud. The concept of the Markov blanket[38] was introduced in the context of Bayesian networks or graphs and referred to as interconnected sets.[39] They provide a statistical way of representing the boundary between an adaptive agent or organism and the world. The underlying mathematics gets complicated and combines contemporary statistics/probability theory, information theory and entropy to explain how an organism can survive in the universe's chaos. Solms calls it a 'statistical concept that separates two groups of states, namely into states inside and outside the system, with the external states separated from those inside the system'.[40] He compares it elsewhere to a kind of membrane separating the inner and outer states of the system. Physically, it lies at the origin of a viewpoint and the possibility of subjectivity that can accompany it.[41] Thanks to self-organisation, the inner world becomes a representative display of what is happening in the outer world. Since free energy acts entropically and thus poses an existential threat to the system, any living thing must minimise this free energy. The drive measures the binding work, and the system or organism learns from experience along the way. Solms transposes this to a task for psychoanalytic science:[42] our predictive models of how the mind works make it more effective and increase the chances of survival and reproduction of our discipline!

Surprising!

By his admission, it took Solms many years to understand that everything revolves around Friston's free energy. *The* eye-opener for him was an article by Carhart-Harris and Friston,[43] which argued that Freud's concept of drive or psychic energy is compatible with the free-energy principle.[44] It hit Solms between the eyes. If mental energy is consistent with thermodynamic free energy, it is measurable and can be captured in physical laws! Note that this is a fundamentally anti-reductionist premise because these formal laws govern the brain and the mind. To Friston, even everything we call mental is mathematically translatable and can be reduced to physical processes of a thermodynamic (entropic versus negentropic forces) and statistical-mechanical (the Markov blanket)[45] kind. His free-energy principle says that any self-organising system in equilibrium with its environment must minimise its free energy for economic reasons.[46] The principle is a mathematical formulation of how adaptive systems (i.e. biological agents, such as animals or brains) resist a natural tendency to disorder.[47] I reproduce some of what he calls critical points from Friston's seminal text here.

Adaptive agents must have limited states and limit the long-term average of surprises to counteract the tendency for disorder/dissolution/entropy to increase. Surprise relies on predictions of sensations, and these predictions rely on an internally generated worldview. Through (Bayesian) probability theory, predictions are encoded. Motor action is directed (and adjusted) by perceptual and proprioceptive feedback. Value is inversely proportional to surprise/free energy for adaptive agents.

For self-organising systems (living ones included) to exist, they must resist entropy by minimising free energy. They must maintain preferred states instead of dissipating in all possible directions. Essential to this is the core theme of optimisation. What is being optimised? Value (expected reward, expected utility) is maximised, or its opposite surprise (*prediction error*, expected cost) is minimised. All this should lead to the most error-free prediction machine possible.

The free-energy principle states that survival is striving to avoid being too surprised by the future. Knowing what might happen is a good survival strategy. Karl Friston understands by life everything capable of predicting its future. From cells to our brains, all are wrapped in (an accumulation of) Markov blankets and sent out to battle the unknown. It is enlightening to describe organisms in this way. Action, perception and learning all become mathematically well-defined properties of the system. Perception provides information to optimise future predictions. Efforts help us escape uncertain (dangerous) situations, and learning is about updating internal states and ideas about the external world. This may seem a very abstract way of looking at things, but those who invoke the Markov blanket see it as a general framework that can be applied to bees as easily as to babies. Of course, this does not mean babies are also like bees.

The essence of homeostasis is that living organisms can only function within a limited spectrum of physical states: the viable, optimal or preferred states or all the states Friston collectively calls the 'expected' states. Our feelings take over when they are absent, and a certain degree of unpredictability arises. We continuously receive information about our likely survival by asking questions about our natural state concerning what is happening around us. How are you? The more uncertain the answers are (i.e. the more information they contain), the worse for us.[48] Solms summarises all this in a one-liner: consciousness arises as a result of surprise, and it is felt uncertainty.

After all this, Solms arrives at a complete reworking of Freud's *Project*, updating the original almost sentence by sentence with the help of current neuroscientific knowledge. Most important errata/addenda that Solms notes are the following.[49] Freud's energy quantum is replaced by free energy: the amount of energy in a system that does not yet provide useful help. Information-theoretically, unpredictability is introduced as the equivalent of entropy in physics. Biologically, the main objective of homeostasis is to resist entropy or increase predictability. Homeostasis underlies Freud's inertia principle of neurons.

Furthermore, Freud's concept of the contact barrier[50] is linked to consolidation/reconsolidation, whereby deeper/earlier predictions are less plastic/changeable than later ones. Stimulus is replaced by *prediction error*, where cognitive processes only begin with incorrect predictions. Freud's conception of bound excitations (vehicles for secondary process thinking and random action) is equated with the buffering function of working memory. According to Miller's law, it can only hold seven to nine bits of information and this only for fifteen to thirty seconds. The reason for this is physiological, as it has to do with the depletion of transmitters.[51] So they have to be used sparingly (through automation). Free-floating excitations (the vehicle of the primary process) are equated with automated responses or non-declarative memory. Freud's systemic consciousness is replaced by precision modulation and the optimisation of predictions. Thus, for another sample of Solms' 'finishing the job' (at least of Freud's psychology as a natural science).[52]

Endnotes

1 Tzara (1975, p. 379).
2 Damasio (1994, 1999, 2018), Panksepp and David (2018), Merker (2007).
3 Hume (2003 [1739]).
4 Chalmers (1995a, 1995b, 2022).

5 Nagel (1974, p. 439). In his paper, he says the subjective nature of consciousness means objective or reductionist methods may continue to come up short in explaining satisfactorily. How to understand the bat's echolocation? Without having a bat's complete mindset and experiences, we don't know what it is to be a bat.

6 Jackson (2002 [1986]).

7 Kihlstrom (1996).

8 Bargh and Chartrand (1999).

9 In his posthumous publication, Bion (1992, p. 38) speaks of an undersea continent he believes produces the unconscious with its alpha function/dream labour (ibid., p. 71).

10 Solms (2021d, p. 158).

11 Damasio (1999).

12 Solms (2021d, pp. 64–65).

13 Teuber (1955).

14 Moruzzi and Magoun (1949).

15 Merker (2007).

16 Solms (2021d, p. 91).

17 Ibid., p. 147.

18 Ibid., p. 150.

19 Ibid., p. 166.

20 According to Björn Merker, it forms the affective-sensory-motor pivot or interface of the brain's 'decision triangle' (Solms, 2021d).

21 For Panksepp, this primal self is the ultimate source of our subjective, sentient being. See Alcaro, Carta, & Panksepp (2017).

22 Solms (2021e, p. 1081).

23 Solms (2013a, 2017c).

24 Freud (1933).

25 Freud (1905a, 1905b) was concerned with oral, anal, phallic or genital drives and their respective objects. To him, these are components of the sexual drive to be distinguished from the Ego or self-preservative drives. Panksepp's typology talks about seven emotional-instinctive systems acting in mutual alloy as (partial) drives.

26 For *The Cambridge Declaration on Consciousness*, see https://fcmconference.org/img/CambridgeDeclarationOnConsciousness.pdf (2012)

27 Hartmann (1951), Solms (2021).

28 Freud (1923a, 1923b).

29 Object relations is an ugly psychoanalytic term for our relationships with others (even when their images have come to inhabit our psyche to a greater or lesser extent).

30 Solms (2021d, p. 171).

31 Ibid., p. 173.

32 Solms and Friston (2018).

33 Solms (2021d, p. 182).

34 Solms (2021e, p. 1056).

35 Ibid., note 19.

36 Friston (2013).

37 Ashby (1962).

38 For the Markov blanket, see Kirchhoff et al. (2018) and see later in this book.

39 Friston (2013).

40 Solms (2021, p. 197).

41 Solms (2021e, p. 1058).

42 Ibid., p. 1061.

43 Carhart-Harris and Friston (2010, 2012).

44 Solms (2021d, p. 180), Carhart-Harris and Friston (2010).

45 Solms (2021d, p. 198).

46 Ibid., p. 10.
47 Friston (2010, p. 127).
48 Solms (2021d, p. 192).
49 Solms (2020).
50 The contact barrier situates itself between preconscious and unconscious. It is a permeable membrane formed from proto-mental elements formed in *joint venture* with the mother (as the most classic first big Other) as *the stuff that dreams* (and thinking) *can be made of*.
51 Solms (2021).
52 Solms (2013b, pp. 389–391).

Chapter 12

Interlude

Psychoanalytic Posology

I have been swimming in many psychoanalytic waters through a confluence of circumstances. Theoretically, clinically and also as part of my analyses.[1] I want to advocate a psychoanalytic posology based on these different kinds of inspiration and experience. Posology is the science of drug dosage. In Belgium, this term is well established. Posology specifies a usual and a maximum dosage for each drug. When prescribing, the patient's age, weight, state of health and tolerance to the drug are considered, among other things.

The drug I want to discuss here is psychoanalytic, which is only figuratively speaking, a drug. It considers and acts on the unconscious, transference or resistance. It also attaches specific importance to matters such as (also infantile, pre-genital) sexuality, the housekeeping of pleasure and displeasure, the structuring effect of Oedipus and castration, the oscillation between the schizoid–paranoid and depressive position and so on. It employs the ground rule of free association, which it responds to with free-floating attention, free-floating responsiveness or reverie. In all this, it pursues not so much magical or chemical healing but primarily a 'remedy by the truth'.

New York psychoanalyst Robert Langs makes a polemical distinction between two forms of therapy: truth therapy versus lie therapy.[2] However effective, (literal) drugs are, in a sense, lie therapy. They can significantly improve or alleviate the course of (especially major) psychiatric disorders and their symptoms or complaints. They may even belong to the framework of, and thus be, potential prerequisites for psychotherapy. For example, the psychomotor inhibition in depression or the overwhelming aspect of anxiety can be so paralysing that sufficient reflection only becomes possible with the necessary medication. But everyone understands that these biological aids alone do not change psychological problems. Pharmacotherapy has nothing to do with truth-telling.

Truth-telling is by no means always practised in psychotherapy, either. The famous hypno- and psychotherapist Milton Erickson had a patient in treatment who believed he was Jesus.[3] He led a passive and withdrawn existence and came to nothing. Erickson told him, 'Your father Joseph is a carpenter, so why not take up woodworking?' He got his patient going that way. He uses – like in the martial art aikido – a (psychopathological) movement of the patient to 'floor' the patient.

DOI: 10.4324/9781003394358-12

He does not fight against the delusion but bends it towards a more productive or constructive direction.

Another example is the so-called paradoxical technique. A person with erythrophobia is instructed to blush as hard as possible several times a day for about five minutes. The same phenomenon changes from undesirable to desirable social behaviour, thanks to the therapist's intervention, thus losing its initial function and meaning. This kind of assistance does have its value. If it allows you to prevent someone from taking their own life, you have, according to many, treated someone effectively.

However, the characteristic of the psychoanalytic forms of treatment is that, in a winged formulation of Michel Thys, they aim at a betterment by truth.[4] Betterment (and I deliberately decline to say what this means) is not pursued magically or chemically. Moreover, the 'good' that the psychoanalytic approach envisions is not life as merely biological but as primarily existential.

According to Wilfred Bion, psychic health would consist primarily in 'suffering the process of thinking': experiencing and containing mental pain rather than getting rid of it in all possible and impossible ways.[5] Paraphrasing Bion, we need truth as much as we need food or oxygen. We cannot, however, breathe it in its pure form.

The framework is the set of arrangements and rules distinguishing ordinary (social) conversation from extraordinary (special) conversation. The framework is the enabling condition for therapy. Like all other forms of psychoanalytic treatment, the classical cure uses its framework, which it applies rather inflexibly. However, many therapies allow the ratio of supporting and discovering elements in the technique to vary according to the patient and the moment of treatment.

The therapeutic relationship is called isomorphic or formally similar to the parent–child relationship. It is asymmetrical and characterised by very different rights and duties. It is the carrier and matrix par excellence of insight and change. The interpretation of the relationship and the relationship itself are the two pillars on which any psychoanalytic treatment rests. The choice of framework prescribed by the psychoanalyst makes a substantial difference.

Returning to posology, the psychoanalytic remedy is not about the calendar age but the mental age of the patient. Where and when are the points of fixation located? This estimation is necessary for good attunement. After all, there is a huge difference in communicating with a baby, a toddler, a primary-school child, an adolescent, a young adult or an adult. What are the duration and frequency of these contacts, and in what environment and in what way do they take place?

Psychoanalytic posology also bases itself on the weight, not of the patient but of the problems. Which elements weigh more heavily than others? How heavy a burden, how much frustration or how many side effects can the patient bear and endure? What about digestion? What lies heavy on the stomach and causes belching? What does the patient 'have on his liver', as in the Dutch saying, meaning: what is bothering the patient that prevents him from or enables him in detoxifying himself? If we are psychoanalysts at heart, should we not also be concerned with excretory functions?

For a long time, psychoanalytic forms of treatment were mainly about indication. The question was: who qualifies for which form of help? I have always reversed this reasoning. How can we offer the patient something psychoanalytic? After all, who does not benefit from the truth? The question then becomes: to which posology can we administer psychoanalytic medicine? Truth must always be mixed with less noble components. Here and there, additions may even be necessary, which need not change anything about truth's power of salvation or efficacy. On the contrary, if there is any form of psychic assistance that considers everyone's uniqueness, it is psychoanalytic. One size fits all? Forget it! Psychoanalysis is not about *prêt-à-porter*/ready-to-wear. It is about *haute couture*/high fashion.

Endnotes

1 Kinet (2013).
2 Langs (1982).
3 Erickson (1992).
4 Thys (2006).
5 Vermote (2018).

Chapter 13

Clinical Neuropsychoanalysis

The Clinical Situation

Concerning the clinic, I quote Solms: 'Neuroscience is no more the final court of appeal for psychoanalysis than psychoanalysis is for neuroscience. The final court of appeal for psychoanalysis is the clinical situation'.[1] Underlying this clinical thinking is the therapeutic relationship with the person suffering (= etymology of 'patient') psychologically. Establishing and maintaining this relationship, for better or worse, is an art and a skill. It requires commitment and attachment, bearing and tolerating, boundaries and understanding. The therapist is not a technologist based on whose prescription the patient is treated but (s)he explores with, around and within each unique patient the always shadowy and complex roots of evil. The Evil from Charles Baudelaire's *Les Fleurs du Mal*[2] is the Evil that implies the dimension of pain above all. Diagnostic is a tentative process leading only to preliminary working hypotheses that never (fully) cover the truth, and therapy is a shared responsibility and enterprise in which the patient does much himself (but not on his own) and the outcome of which cannot be guaranteed (and certainly not exactly).[3]

In this clinical situation, the psychoanalytic therapist suspends his knowledge. Under the motto 'throw away the book', he cleverly keeps himself dumb, shrouds himself in a learnt ignorance or *docta ignorantia* and respectfully gives way to the knowledge hidden in the patient's unconscious. It can only be read in and between the lines of the book our patient opens with us. Any a priori knowledge on the therapist's part (be it psychiatric or psychoanalytic, Lacanian or neuropsychoanalytic) can impede the burgeoning unconscious understanding hidden inside the patient. The basic rule of free association thus leads to the patient telling what he would not tell anyone else (himself included). Ultimately, little human is alien to either the patient or the psychotherapist. Or indeed: even little *inhuman* is alien to them. From what he knows about how the human mind works, the psychoanalyst wants to help the patient move forward by becoming better through the truth. With a midwife as a mother, Socrates already developed this maieutic or midwifery method, in a sense, (only) helping to discover what was hidden in his interlocutor's knowledge. In Socrates' view, knowledge is, in a way, recollection. He would sometimes compare himself to a hornet preventing the winged horse Pegasus from ascending to heaven. I like the analogy of the psychoanalyst as a court jester. Only

DOI: 10.4324/9781003394358-13

through his 'funny talk' does His Majesty the 'Ego' allow himself to be knocked off his throne from time to (appropriate) time.

All this remains true to this day in the psychoanalytic therapy of neuroses. Paul Verhaeghe speaks of psychopathology, and Peter Fonagy of representational mental disorders in this context.[4] In their symbolic-imaginary hypertrophy, the analytic task relies mainly on the ability to 'cut the crap'. This deconstruction contributes to seeking or inventing other balances. By contrast, symbolic-imaginary hypotrophy exists in actual pathology or mental process disorders. Evacuation of mental content prevails over mentalisation, drive-, affect- and emotion-regulation problems are predominant; a secure basis and an adequately equipped mental apparatus are lacking. Freud's comparison between the working method of the sculptor (*per via de levare*) and that of the painter (*per via di porre*) remains pertinent here.[5] In the former, the sculpture is already present in the marble; it only needs to be liberated from it. In the latter, shape and colour are added to the canvas layer by layer and brushstroke by brushstroke. Construction rather than deconstruction is then in the zenith. All this is inspired not in the least by what (also intraverbal and affectively) comes live on stage in the therapeutic relationship.

If we translate to the clinical situation all that has been said in this book until now, it seems necessary that the patient will be surprised or disturbed during his psychotherapy. This is no doubt why psychoanalytic therapies are sometimes called '*anxiety-provoking*'.[6] Some authors go so far as to allude to the violence of interpretation or compare interpretation to the enigmatic *koan* of a Zen master.[7] For example: listen to the clapping of one hand. But let us keep both feet firmly on Western soil because psychoanalytic efficacy requires significantly more than one-off highs. First, I will briefly recapitulate some general clinical principles we can derive from Solms' neuropsychoanalysis. I will also present some of his views on psychopathology.[8] Primarily based on the article mentioned above on the scientific standing of psychoanalysis and neurobiologically detailed elaboration of it,[9] I will provide some of his psychotherapeutic recommendations. They may not contain much new to the clinician, but they read like a powerful *oratio pro domo* for Solms' trajectory and project.

Above all, from a neuroscientific angle, they confirm a psychoanalytic essence, as it was summarised in one sentence by former president of the *International Psychoanalytical Association* Horacio Etchegoyen: 'Psychoanalysis is a method that recognises the past in the present and distinguishes it through interpretation'.[10] After over a century of work in consulting rooms worldwide, psychoanalytic findings are confirmed or falsified for once from another perspective (in an allusion to Karl Popper's critique of psychoanalysis as a pseudoscience). This also immediately addresses a significant complaint of neuropsychoanalyst *avant-la-lettre* (and teacher of Ariane Bazan) Howard Shevrin.[11]

Neuropsychoanalysis in the Clinic

Neuropsychoanalysis focuses mainly on our emotional life. We saw that for Solms, our feelings ultimately stem from our Id. They let us know how we are. Ideally, however, our Ego is not only guided by these feelings but also by the reality principle. The Ego pursues as much automation as possible to save energy. In other words, there is pressure for long-term or non-declarative memory consolidation. Our working memory, aka *short-term memory*, is, therefore, minimal. We should only become aware of something when necessary, namely when we trip over something or fall. We can, then, quote James Joyce:[12] (exceptionally with good reason) 'Mistakes are the portals of discovery'. Consciousness is, therefore (with a nod to Werner Heisenberg)[13] based on the uncertainty principle. Like Joseph LeDoux's two (different speeds of the) fear systems, conscious/secondary processes are slow and unconscious/primary fast. In precarious life situations, haste is imperative, and procrastination is dangerous. Subcortical structures immediately seize the wheel. They direct, rule and react.

Meanwhile, the Ego learns from experience, and frequent updating and reconsolidation occurs. Too much detailed consideration of the various memory systems in the brain is beyond our current scope. I am happy to refer to world authorities on the subject, namely Daniel Schacter,[14] Douwe Draaisma[15] or a more recent review by Alvor Pastor.[16] I am only reviewing some broad outlines relevant to the subject matter discussed here. Some forms of learning are rapid – for example, emotional or *single-exposure learning*. Solms always gives the same example in his lectures: you only put your fingers in an electrical socket once. After that, you never do it again. Even a single sexual can leave lasting traces also. Using Ariane Bazan's reasoning, I will explain this later on. Then again, learning that has to do with attachment takes many months. All the memories/predictions we retain from the beginning of our life end up in non-declarative/implicit memory. They are hard to learn and hard to forget. They cannot be reconsolidated through awareness but only by experience. Freud calls this the most laborious and lengthy component of psychoanalytic work, *working through*. It is learning by repetition and by (inter-)acting.[17] Similarly, an inevitable drudgery outside the consulting room and in real life during the psychoanalytic process need not necessarily be considered enactment or acting out[18] but can signify a form of *per-agir* or acting through.[19]

We are not born a *tabula rasa* but are evolutionarily pre-wired. While pharmacotherapy acts chemically on emotional-instinctive systems, therapeutic change involves changing predictions. We saw that, according to Solms, the cortex stabilises/binds consciousness (cf his *mental solids*) but *does not* generate it. The cortical level binds affective arousal and transforms it into conscious cognition. To clarify these processes, Solms repeatedly paraphrases a statement made by Freud in *Beyond the Pleasure Principle*: instead of consciousness, a memory trace appears. This process is called consolidation, and the reverse movement (instead of a memory trace, consciousness appears) is then called reconsolidation.[20] Consolidation is reversed/undone at that point. The memory trace is dissolved. It becomes *salient/activated* again and therefore unstable and susceptible to both revision and reconsolidation. Solms calls this reconsolidating work 'predictive work in progress'.[21]

Paraphrasing Freud, the world is not a nursery. If we were (sufficiently) lucky, our parents ran ragged, taking care of all our needs. They liked seeing us as (if we were) an extension of themselves and surrounded us with loving attention (nowadays: TLC or tender loving care). We then fell like Obelix[22] into a vat of magic potion that strengthened us for the rest of our lives. Apart from the people we love and who love us, the outside world is largely indifferent to us for the rest of our lives. The fact that our needs and desires can only be met in this outer world makes life so difficult. One cannot very well have sex with or attach oneself to oneself (although psychoanalytic theories on narcissism show we can try). The primary developmental task is learning how to get by in the outside world. After all, it is not *l'art pour l'art*. We learn not *to* learn but mainly to install optimal predictions about how we best succeed in a particular environment. Freud[23] calls all this the development of the Ego or, in his famous one-liner: *Wo Es war soll Ich werden*.[24]

Most of our predictions are carried out unconsciously. Innate/instinctive predictions take effect automatically. So do those acquired roughly in our famous 'first thousand days' before the preconscious/declarative/explicit/hippocampal memory system has matured. It is the period of infantile amnesia, which Freud said was due to the repression of the Oedipal, but which correlates in every way with the afore-mentioned neurobiological findings. Infantile amnesia does, however, apply only to episodic and semantic memory.[25] There are several unconscious/non-declarative/implicit memory systems but the most important ones for psychopathology are procedural[26] and emotional, each operating according to its principles. They both go beyond reason (hence Freud's repetition compulsion - see below), and they define the functioning mode of the unconscious system.

We learn to solve our problems permanently, and to the extent that we achieve this goal, preconscious predictions are consolidated and reconsolidated more deeply. Neurally, this implies that they are transferred from cortical to subcortical memory systems. Solms localised Freud's preconscious in the cortex and the systemic unconscious in the *basal ganglia* and *cerebellum*.[27] However, the cognitive unconscious differs from the dynamic unconscious within the systemic unconscious. The former is also called the unconscious Ego insofar as it lacks the psychodynamic processes characterising what was repressed. Repression is preceded by/derived from cognitive (represented) processes and learning, while the Id is endogenous and consists of affective (and non-represented) processes.

Psychotherapy

It is crucial to remember that these are unrepresented or (perhaps better) unimaginable programmes of action. Therefore, they cannot be 'retrieved' by working memory either. Truly unconscious (as opposed to preconscious) memories cannot be updated within conscious/working memory. In this sense, they are both indelible and highly operative. Joseph LeDoux's model distinguished between the 'high road' and the 'low road', where incoming stimuli from the thalamus are sent on the one hand to the (slower) neocortex and on the other to the faster *amygdala* for rational and emotional processing, respectively. The latter proceeds, in his terms, 'quick and dirty'[28] and forms the neural basis of what Freud calls the primary process.[29]

All this does not mean non-declarative memories would not be amenable to processing. It *does* mean that cognition/thinking is not enough but must be accompanied by experience. Non-declarative memories become activated and editable only through an embodied event, namely by discussing non-declarative memory traces through their derivatives in the here and now (hence the importance of transference interpretations).[30] The non-declarative predictions cannot be incorporated into working memory, but patients can be made aware that these predictions come *live on stage* when repeated in endless variations. Given sufficient repeated and interpretive editing, they ultimately die like a fugue. Both learning and unlearning require repetition. For Solms, this is the essence of the psychoanalytic cure.[31]

To Solms, the distinction between the descriptive/cognitive and the dynamic unconscious finally rests in the following. The cognitive unconscious consists of predictions that were legitimately or rightly automated. They are deeply ingrained precisely because they work so well. They succeed in both long-term and reliable ways of attending to underlying needs. By contrast, what has been repressed was wrongly (or prematurely) automated. This happens when the Ego is overwhelmed by difficulties. The Ego then needs help figuring out how to satisfy the imperatives of the Id in the external world. Of course, this happens most often in childhood, when our Ego is still weak and underdeveloped. The child tries to repress/forget and, to this end, automates the best (often more or less wish-fulfilling) predictions of the moment. It simply tries to 'make the best' of a difficult job.

For predictions to be corrected or fine-tuned as a function of experience, they must be reconsolidated. Memory traces must give way to consciousness so long-term memory can become labile again. However, according to Solms, this is difficult with repression because it is immune to (declarative) reconsolidation despite repetitive fear/prediction errors. Although automated prediction does not work, it is considered (in a sense, against its better judgement) that it *does* work. The Ego prefers that problems can be regarded as solved rather than unsolved. Freud calls this resistance, and it triggers defence mechanisms. We prefer to confirm our predictions rather than *dis*confirm them. Solms refers to the famous confirmation bias or self-serving bias.[32] Fear or prediction error testifies to the constant (pressure of the imminent) return of what was repressed against which we defend ourselves using all kinds of after-repression.[33] Additional defence mechanisms must then be deployed,[34] or else all sorts of means will be used in the service of defence.[35]

I often quote French author E.M. Cioran : *'Ce n'est pas par le génie, c'est par la souffrance, par elle seule, qu'on cesse d'être une marionnette'*.[36] Only suffering can free us from determinism (or automatism). Using reason, we can free ourselves from who or what pulls the strings. In the psychoanalytic process, we analyse what the patient cannot cope with. Together, we try to understand in what possible and impossible ways he has tried to help himself. Patterns and automatisms installed over the years must be replaced (always after much jolting, trial and error) by new ways the patient has to make or pave for himself. For consolation, Goethe's famous motto may safely be kept in mind in this regard: *'Und so lang du das nicht hast,/Dieses: stirb und werde,!/Bist du nur ein trüber Gast/Auf der dunklen Erde'*[37] ('And as long you don't have that/This: Die and become!/You're only a gloomy guest/On the dark earth'.)

For a long time, the psychoanalytic technique focused mainly on insight and interpretation. It particularly appealed to declarative memory and life histories that could be put into words. When this failed, it was blamed on repression. However, many experiences were never recorded in episodic memory, which depends on an operational *hippocampus*. They were pre- or infra-verbal or traumatising experiences. Indeed, the latter disrupt the functioning of the *hippocampus*.[38] Paradoxically, there is also hypermnesia or memory compulsion[39] characterising post-traumatic stress disorder, in which all kinds of somatosensory sensations remain etched, as it were, on the retina and other membranes.

It is peculiar to psychoanalytic therapy that feelings need to be understood (rather than chemically influenced), and that deeply automated predictions need to be changed. Which feelings prevail? How can they (indirectly) be inferred from feelings, sensitivities or behaviour? Since we mostly try to satisfy our emotional needs unconsciously, we must first become aware of them to change them.[40] Given that non-declarative memory is unforgettable or indelible and that repression causes resistance to the reappearance of conflicts that were deemed unresolvable, reconsolidation is a difficult task. It requires prolonged treatment with sufficient repetition and at a sufficiently high frequency for development to be possible.

Oedipus Complex and Sexuality

In 2019 I co-edited the book *Triangular Relationships: Current Oedipal Variations*, in which the Oedipus complex is tested against contemporary theory and clinic. Classically Freudian, the Oedipus complex is the core complex of neurosis.[41] Our identity and relationships are grouped around it. It is supposed to be decisive to our gender and sexual orientation and the formation of our conscience as civilised human beings. For Andre Green,[42] the Oedipus complex provides an initial and foundational symbolic structure. It has varying manifestations depending on time and place and is embodied by different figures and with different functions. In Lacanian terms, the great Other takes root in our unconscious and turns us into a '*zoön politikon*' or political animal.[43] After all, the family cannot be reduced to biological affinities but is a configuration, varying in time and culture, of interrelationships, commandments and prohibitions, rights and duties, not least in terms of who may 'enjoy' what, from whom and how.

Let us look at the clinical situation. For the optimal psychosocial and -sexual development of the child, the parent's love for each other is usually more important than the parent's love for the child. If the parents have an unsatisfactory relationship, a lopsided triangle can develop, with one or both parents seeking gratification from the child. The child is thus not sufficiently confronted with loving parents in a sexual couple. The child seems to connect with the mother or the father more than the partner does and thinks it can or should satisfy their desires. The boundaries between the sexes, between the generations, and the boundaries related to incest then become unclear. What falls short here is the paternal function (not to be confused with the father as a figure), which as a third term, should prohibit *and* protect.

Typically, it thus curbs the boundless love in which parent and child merge in pathological or fatal ways. These are mainly universal desires, in which the child must be lovingly put or kept 'in place' to install a proper triangle. When this triangulation functions appropriately, the child is confronted with boundaries and with desires of which it is *not* the centre. Therefore, this process has a protective value. It prevents the child from getting stuck, fixated and thus impaired in its psychosexual development and individuation.

Taking this Oedipus complex as an example, Solms points out that we can never remember wanting to go to bed with one parent and get rid of the other. This configuration only looms large from later (also symbolic or imaginary) enactment and repetition of patterns throughout our (love- and other) lives. For instance, one repeatedly gets mixed up in amorous or sexual triangulations or other imbroglios. There are frequently forbidden/impossible loves that (guilt: *must!*) end badly. By dwelling on this and reflecting on it, the gaze is opened and only by wielding the psychotherapeutic iron for a sufficiently long and intense period can 'false' folds be more or less smoothed out or replaced by other and more realistic predictions.

Solms cites the Oedipus complex as a prime example of an unsolvable problem. If you want to monopolise one parent, you must eliminate the other. Don't the dilemmas resulting from such violently conflicting tendencies embrace an inevitable and, for the child, unsolvable constellation of mutually clashing emotions? The child must cut many Oedipal knots without much know-how to avoid endlessly faltering on an inextricable problem. At least they can then use their energy (and working memory capacity) to tackle the issues and tasks they *can* solve. But cutting knots is not the same as resolving or untangling them, so that later in life, the return of what was repressed is more the rule than the exception.

In his recent reworking of the Oedipus complex, Solms[44] refutes the phylogenetic slant that Freud[45] had developed. Freud still considered castration anxiety, horror in the face of incest and guilt as phylogenetic legacies. This was in line with Jean-Baptiste Lamarck's assumption, still widely accepted in Freud's time, whereby acquired traits would be inherited. All memory research completely contradicts these inherited memories.[46] In contrast, Solms holds all the mutually clashing and intense emotions the child inevitably experiences towards his first love objects responsible for the Oedipus complex.[47] I quote: 'It arises from the unavoidably competing demands of the six basic emotional needs that every child must learn to master within the confines of the family it is born into. These six basic needs are innate, but the Oedipus complex is not.[48] In all this reasoning, it is unsurprising that Solms assigns a leading role to PLAY, particularly in developing the Oedipus complex. To Solms, psychological maturity is also not linked to some 'classical' or 'normal' settlement of the Oedipus complex. The highest settlement achievable is a good-enough reconciliation of the various drive requirements. It is not about the hetero-normative but rather about achieving Melanie Klein's depressive position.[49] It is noteworthy, however, that any reference to the law or the paternal function is absent from Solms' discussion of the Oedipus complex. This while the *Non* and the *Nom-du-Père* (the No and the Name-of-the-Father- particularly in Lacan's return to Freud) play a vital role in the Oedipus complex. Also, sexuality is by no means given the leading role that was attributed to it by Freud.

Not only the drive, the energetic-economic perspective or Freud's neuroscientific roots have fallen into the background within psychoanalysis. This is equally true of sexuality, virtually absent from (object-)relational psychoanalysis and post-Kleinian thought.[50] In connection with Winnicott, Adam Philips speaks succinctly of a flight from the erotic.[51] With Solms, too, it is no longer given the leading role assigned to it by Freud. To him, LUST seems to be just one of the emotional instincts alongside others. In contrast, to Freud, the distinction between the sexual and the Ego- or self-preservative drives was still essential, and they have separate fates. The sexual drive lends itself foremost to all kinds of symbolic-imaginary processing and sublimation. Until now, the polymorphously perverse disposition of the child introduced by Freud in his *Three Essays on the Theory of Sexuality* or perversion as a separate structure elaborated by Lacan seems to have disappeared entirely in Solms' neuropsychoanalysis ...

Even in the index of the landmark publication *Affect Regulation, Mentalisation and the Development of the Self*,[52] sexuality is still conspicuous by its absence. In this book, Peter Fonagy and his colleagues describe at length that the 'mirroring of affect' plays a central role in developing the capacity for mentalisation. Repeated external mirroring by the mother of what the child experiences have a substantial 'educational' function.[53] Such mirroring results in a growing ability to correctly identify the internal arousal belonging to this or that specific emotional category in which the infant finds itself.[54] At the same time, the small child develops an ability to attribute to itself the information associated with this emotion. This enables it to both imagine and predict the behaviour they commonly exhibit in this state.[55] The mirroring referred to here is a critical learning process with adaptive significance.

In a later publication, however, they argue that this mirroring does *not* occur where it concerns sexual emotions. Here, the (m-)other looks away. She appears incapable of mirroring. This, according to Fonagy, makes sexuality both unique and problematic. In taking this position, he aligns himself in specific ways with Jean Laplanche's theory of general seduction when he argues that the child is inevitably traumatised by unconscious enigmatic sexual signifiers of the mother. Indeed, child observations suggest that child sexual arousal (quite unlike other emotions) is not mirrored but ignored, too little 'marked' or even incongruously mirrored. Sexuality does not become mentalised because, according to Fonagy, in sexual matters, we all remain more or less borderline. I quote: 'Sexual arousal can never truly be experienced as owned. It will always be an imposed burden'.[56]

We struggle with and also freak out over the *crazy little thing* (not called love but) *called sex*. Even in later life, the child feels that it encounters a taboo regarding sexuality. Sex seems a somewhat secretive and forbidden domain. Whether the woman wears a bikini or a burka: in any case, there is nudity that must not be seen under any circumstances. The child is also confronted with adults who suddenly start acting weird as soon as it comes to sexual body parts or activities. Are they dirty, then? Are they not allowed to be seen? Why are they accompanied by excitement so tricky to understand? How different is it from the 'make love not war' of bonobos who, like humans, use sex to deepen relationships, comfort each other, have fun or experience pleasure? They do this without embarrassment, guilt or shame, or shall we say without any (Oedipus or other) complexes?[57]

Solms as Psychopathologist

A hypertrophy of its prefrontal lobes succinctly characterises Homo sapiens. The massive increase in the human neocortex is thought to be mainly caused by the duplication of a single gene (ARHGAP118).[58] It enables us to inhibit and think (ideationally).[59] Our animal brothers and sisters also possess these capabilities but are much more limited. The prefrontal cortex is the furthest removed from the external sensorimotor periphery and our deeper bodily viscera. It contains highly abstract sets of algorithms that, in the broad sense, are linguistically structured. This is linked to our capacity for symbolic communication and legislative work, both of which order our living (together). However, these specific human achievements have a downside: we still need to be made aware of what drives or moves us emotionally. What are we doing and why? We make up all kinds of stories to lend meaning to our actions. Ultimately, we either believe our fabrications or regard them as gospel set in stone. At worst, we start a more or less Holy War on their behalf.

Going back to the beginning, the difference between neurology and psychiatry is not between (anatomical) structure and (psychological) function but between varied observational perspectives. It is about the distinction between *having* a brain and *being* a brain. A nomothetic and general human perspective prevails in the former, and in the latter, an ideographic and individual view. For the treatment of your multiple sclerosis or your Parkinson's disease, you go to the neurologist. Still, with what it means to you to be a human being with multiple sclerosis or Parkinson's, you should (at least in principle) be better off with a psychiatrist.

Being a brain (our *mind*) springs from a network of brain circuits, each with particular functions. The most important two are consciousness and intentionality. We saw that at the basis of consciousness is the pleasure/unpleasure principle. It is associated with the PAG. Our intentionality, on the other hand, can be divided into seven major components, each of which is linked to primary emotions: (1) curiosity and interest, (2) consumption and pleasure, (3) joy and play, (4) care and love, (5) panic and grief, (6) terror and fear, (7) anger and rage. Each has its specific neurophysiology and is vital in universally recognisable life situations. It is, therefore, not surprising that the various psychopharmaceuticals act on these same circuits. These emotional systems underlie both our mental functioning and its problems. They are individualised according to life history. They become more or less regulated by frontal structures that evolve in a very experience-dependent way and only fully mature once we are in our twenties. This neuroplasticity is responsible for the socio-cultural dimension of psychological problems. It is also at the origin of our capacity for *agency* or, as the case may be, our so-called free will.

The epigenetic influences, in particular, require the special attention of psychiatry. We probably all know our mums and dads (or other important characters who figured in our childhood stage) are essential. Pre-eminently, psychoanalysis makes clear and understandable how great, comprehensive, and haunting their influence on our mental life is.

In his 2019 clinical lectures, Solms[60] uses several principles I wholeheartedly share (especially as a psychiatrist-psychoanalyst, often confronted with patients who seek help but not psychoanalysis). The question he poses there (*Does one size fit all?*) must be answered with 'no'. I refer to Neville Symington[61] because he explicitly distances himself from anyone 'who disdains to adapt himself to the idiosyncrasies of the individual'. Paraphrasing Wilfred Bion, we need truth like oxygen, but we cannot breathe it in its pure form. Like any medicine, the dose of this truth must be adjusted according to the patient and the moment. In the previous interlude, therefore, I talked about a psychoanalytic posology.

Although Solms recognises the highly valued subtleties and complexities, even the poetry of the consulting room, he compares psychoanalysis more prosaically to medical practice. His bottom line is that a patient (i.e. someone who suffers) seeks help from a (sometimes supposed) expert. According to Solms, all those who ask for help can be helped psychoanalytically. Although not all in the same way. To do so, the psychoanalyst must assess the main problem. The patient may well have both cancer and a bladder infection. Both then deserve care and treatment, but which takes precedence? Solms situates himself within the classical Anglo-Saxon tradition: (post-)Kleinian and object-relational supplemented with a pinch of self-psychology.[62] To him, psychopathology is characterised by three fundamentally different ways of banishing content from our minds: the psychotic, the narcissistic and the neurotic.[63] Each of us may exhibit traits of all three, but only one of them is decisive.

In our ontogeny, we are initially mere bodies. We are born in Id. We are all needs and dependencies and don't know anything yet. We do have emotional instincts that are evolutionarily ready, but we have yet to learn everything about how reality (including socio-cultural reality) works. I like to compare it to Aristotle's distinction between *techne* and *episteme*. A bird or a craftsman has *techne* and can make a nest or furniture without being aware of the laws (*episteme*) governing a rectangular triangle. At the outset, our mindset is that of the primary process and an excellent way to satisfy (especially our emotional) drives is hallucinatory wish fulfilment. It is the stage of primary narcissism in which you can delude yourself into anything. If this mode still prevails even in adulthood, you are in the psychotic register, where the Id reigns, and reality is rejected. Indeed, in psychosis, the patient's Ego turns away from the outside world to make way for an omnipotent creation of a delusional and/or hallucinatory nature. In his lectures, Solms is very formal in this: after all, who better than he know the psychoses that so often prevail in neurological patients...? Solms does draw from a very classical Freudian and psychiatric perspective regarding psychoses. That there are addenda and errata to be added from both (post-) Kleinian and Lacanian quarters, however, is a subject for many other books.[64]

While after our birth, the Id is still entirely in control, the Ego (rudimentarily present or *in statu nascendi* at first) begins to learn what works and what does not, and it builds up representations/memories/predictions. Thus, more and more realism develops. What is positive we absorb, and what is negative we spit out. For survival, the distinction between friend and foe is vital, and the former must be protected/shielded from the latter. Splitting is an adaptive achievement that allows us to approach what is good for us and avoid what harms us. We are immediately at a narcissistic level, caught between a primitive and haunting Superego (Melanie Klein)[65] and an Ideal Ego (Freud) to which we can never or will never respond. We may try to appropriate suitable objects and exorcise bad ones, but this operation/organisation remains unstable because the split-off (also) returns sooner or later. In the adult, narcissistic pathology occurs when there is insufficient separation between self and object. Good and evil, love and hate remain split and are held far apart within the self or the object. Solms distances himself from (if he is not annoyed by) overly broad use of the term 'psychotic' mechanisms among (post-) Kleinians. Indeed, to him, they are (admittedly schizoid-paranoid, but) essentially narcissistic mechanisms.[66] Unfortunately, Solms' diagnosis of psychoanalysis, which he calls somewhat narcissistic, is also recognisable. Its libido is invested more in itself than in the object or the outside world, it lavishly avails itself of division throughout its movement and finally, according to him, its self-importance of omniscience and omnipotence contrasts with a devaluation of dissenters.

Pretending we can create reality (instead of adapting to it), however, is not very fruitful. Fantasy is beautiful, but it cannot replace the satisfaction that can only be found in reality. In cases of neurotic problems, the narcissistic Ego is replaced by a more realistic Ego. Objects (even liked, cf. the so-called object love) can be seen as separate from the self. There is grief, loss of omnipotence, vulnerability, smallness and dependence, all characteristic of Melanie Klein's depressive position. In neurotic problems, it is not reality but drive that is sacrificed. You try to push unwanted feelings away first, and then you try also to keep them away from your conscious awareness: repression and after-pressure, respectively. This can lead to the typical character formation (based on reaction formation),[67] but when constriction/inhibition/avoidance does not work (anymore), the exile returns to the scene in disguised form, and the patient suffers from the return of what was repressed, and a symptom arises as a kind of compromise or composite formation. This symptom indicates to us that there is something we cannot get rid of and are trying to banish from our consciousness. Apart from repression and pursuing this repression (using additional defensive troops and tricks), you can also split or cleave, in which case there is a (not horizontal but) *vertical* compartmentalisation in your psyche. Pieces of the self are then regressively banished to an external (projection) or internal (introjection) 'foreign country'. A third and more disastrous 'solution' is to sink back to your earliest stage of development, denying reality and replacing it with delusion.

Solms regards various self-destructive problems so common in the clinical situation (such as the adverse therapeutic reaction, addiction, suicidality or self-mutilation) as ways of achieving immediate gratification without doing the necessary mental work. In Bion's terms, the person avoids *suffering the process of thinking*. They are ways of circumventing the reality principle; in this sense, they are pathological forms of Ego-functioning. He gives the example of how, when abandoned, we do not seek proximity to the love object but immediate gratification from opiates such as morphine or heroin. Here, the relevant neuromodulators (beta-endorphin acting on mu-opioid receptors) are directly 'used' to achieve satisfaction. That this is harmful or destructive is not a result of a supposed death drive but of a failing defence mechanism on the part of the Ego.[68]

Those at home in psychoanalytic practice will likely find little new in all the above. Indeed, after some hundred and twenty-five years of reporting from consulting rooms worldwide, it is *nil novi sub sole*. Nothing new under the sun. However, Solms' Latin is much less hermetic or esoteric, so his (neuro-)psychoanalytic transmitter leads to much better and broader reception, paradoxically perhaps especially *outside* the more narrow psychoanalytic world.

Endnotes

1 Johnson and Flores Mosri (2016, p. 10).
2 Baudelaire (1876).
3 Kinet (2023).
4 Verhaeghe (2002) introduced the spectrum between actual pathology- and psychopathology that can be used within each personality structure (Lacanian: neurotic, perverse, psychotic). It is close to the divide between mental process disorders and mental representational disorders introduced by Fonagy e.a. (2003). The former are about the ability to bear, think or grasp mental content, and the latter is about mental content per se. Actual pathology/mental process disorder is characterised by anxiety against which the subject cannot defend himself. In psychopathology, conversely, a whole arsenal of symptoms is developed as a more or less successful defence against anxiety. Consequently, psychoneurotic fear is less overwhelming or traumatic and is limited by this psychic or symbolic processing. In actual pathology, unbound drive or trauma leads to various rather nonspecific disturbances in physical and mental functioning. The main defence mechanisms here are the flight, evacuation or acting out characterising so many severe personality disorders and in which the patient is most of all in need of a therapist who acts as a mentalising object (with its digestive, metabolising and translating function). In Lacanian terminology, all signification is phallic.
5 In his discussion on Leonardo da Vinci (Freud, 1905a, p. 20).
6 For example, by one of the pioneers of psychoanalytic psychotherapy Peter Sifneos (1992).
7 Aulagnier (2003).
8 Vermote (2018).
9 Solms (2019b): three clinical seminars on YouTube entitled *Does one size fit all?*
10 Solms (2018a, 2018b).
11 Etchegoyen (1999, p. 112).
12 Shevrin (1995).
13 Joyce (2012 [1922]).
14 Werner Heisenberg's uncertainty principle of 1927 is, as it were, the equivalent of Rubin's vase in physics. There are so-called incommensurable pairs of quantities, for which it holds that the values of both quantities cannot be fixed simultaneously.

Examples of such pairs from physics are place and impulse or energy and time. In this neuropsychoanalytic account, they then become nature and mind, subcortical and cortical, and sensation and mind.

15 Schacter (2001).
16 Draaisma (2010).
17 Pastor (2020).
18 Freud (1914a, 1914b).
19 For my more detailed discussion of acting out, see Kinet (1992).
20 Vansina-Cobbaert (1993).
21 'Consciousness arises instead of a memory trace' (Freud 1920b, p. 25). Nader, Schafe and LeDoux (2000), Tronson and Taylor (2007).
22 Solms (2021e, p. 1084).
23 Obelix is a sympathetic and unusually strong character from Asterix, a Belgian-French *bande dessinée* (comic book) series published in over seventy countries and translated into more than a hundred languages. More than 350 million copies have been sold, making Asterix the best-sold series in Europe.
24 Freud (1923a, 1923b).
25 Freud (1933a, 1933b) Lacan plays a lot with this Freudian maxim. One could argue that he turns it around: *Wo Ich war soll Es werden.* That is to say, with Es = S of the subject (of the unconscious). We should not liberate our Ego but free ourselves *from* our (specular) Ego.
26 Episodic memory: anecdotal/narrative/explicit (fragments of) memories. Semantic memory (meaning of terms, words, symbols).
27 We cannot recount how we learnt to ride a bike, swim or play the piano. Memory is expressed in the form of action. Cycling is *hard to learn* but also *hard to forget*. By the way, this is not only true about action but also about interaction (both with ourselves and others).
28 Solms (2017b).
29 LeDoux (1994).
30 Freud (1911a, 1911b).
31 Transference is thought to be related more to procedural and emotional memory (Turnbull et al. 2006).
32 Solms (2018 a, 2018b).
33 Campbell and Sedikides (1999).
34 See Anna Freud's defence mechanisms (1936) again.
35 See earlier note. Some defence mechanisms are imaginary, and we have in common with animals, e.g. fleeing and freezing. Most defence mechanisms are linguistic/symbolic, e.g. displacement and reaction formation.
36 Cioran (1987).
37 From *Selige Sehnsucht* by Johann Wolfgang von Goethe (1999 [1819]). For German and English versions, see https://www.jstor.org/stable/462504
38 Yovell, Solms and Fotopoulou (2015), Flores Mosri (2021).
39 A happy neologism by Thys (2023), as a counterpart to the repetition compulsion.
40 Third core claim of Solms (2018c).
41 Freud (1933b, p. 126).
42 Kinet (1992).
43 Ackrill (1994).
44 Solms (2021f).
45 Freud (1912–1913a, b).
46 Solms (2021f, p. 559).
47 Ibid., p. 571.
48 Ibid.

49 Ibid., p. 572. See also note 11.
50 Fonagy (2008).
51 Phillips (1988, p. 152).
52 Fonagy et al. (2004).
53 Ibid., p. 161.
54 Ibid.
55 Ibid., p. 192.
56 Fonagy (2008, p. 19).
57 Van Coillie (2022), Wrangham and Peterson (1998, p. 198).
58 It is a mere 804 bases long (Florio et al. 2015) in Solms (2021f, p. 562).
59 This ideational thinking is determined by encoding in cortical tissues coordinated primarily by the *hippocampus* i.e. also cortical, though more primitive than the neocortex Solms (2021f, p. 559). Episodic and semantic memories are ideational in nature.
60 Solms (2019a).
61 Symington (1986, p. 193) quotes Sandor Ferenczi (whom he calls the long forgotten (but now restored to honour) innovator of psychoanalysis): *Is it always the patient's resistance that is the cause of failure? Is it not rather our own convenience, which disdains to adapt itself, even in technique, to the idiosyncrasies of the individual?*
62 Self-psychology focuses mainly on our sense of self or self-image, as proprioception or in its specular guise, respectively: the *looking-glass* self. Ego and self are often confused with each other. The former is a supposed mental apparatus, while the self relates more to our imaginary and symbolic identity. Regulating a sense of self and self-esteem is then one of the functions of the Ego. The subject the Lacanians talk about is a *res cogitans* or thinking thing hidden under both and is never (completely) covered by the Ego or the self.
63 This tripartite division can be found in Kernberg (1975) and more recently in McWilliams (2011). Lacanians distinguish the neurotic, the perverse and the psychotic structure characterised by repression, disavowal and rejection.
64 For a broad overview, see Lombardo, Rinaldi and Thanopulos (2019) and from a specifically Lacanian angle Vanheule (2011).
65 Segal (1964) and Kinet (1996).
66 In narcissistic love, the other is a small other: a piece of the self or an other-similar. This narcissistic love is distinguished from object love, where the (love) object (also in its radical alterity cf the big Other) is loved see Kinet (2005).
67 One of the defence mechanisms described by both Father Freud and Daughter Anna Freud is reaction formation. When you act overly friendly or politely towards someone, you can't stand. It is a mechanism that plays a vital role in character formation (often unknowingly).
68 Solms (2021e, p. 1054).

Chapter 14

Interlude

Kent & I

Adoption is a classic in our cultural heritage. Moses, Oliver Twist and Peter Pan are well-known foundlings who were adopted. But adoption also plays a vital role in psychoanalysis. Let us remember that Oedipus grew up as the adopted child of Polybus and Merope. According to Freud, many neurotics cherish adoption as a fantasy. They think they are adopted, and at the same time, they fantasise about their birth parents, who are better, bigger, more prosperous or nobler than those imperfect figures who (only) pretend to be their parents. In this way, they can continue to imagine themselves as descendants of giants, kings and queens and temper their ambivalent feelings by distributing them among different figures. From my (mainly clinical) psychotherapeutic practice, such fantasised and idealised parents appear to be especially prevalent among those who have manifestly grown up in adverse circumstances.

We are born with several expectations to which we believe we are 'naturally' entitled. If they are not met, we feel we have been wronged. It is not only the king-bully Richard III who uses the logic of 'destructive entitlement/right'. I am referring here to a concept of Ivan Boszormenyi-Nagy from contextual therapy: those who feel wronged (usually in a more invisible way than Shakespeare's 'hero') consider themselves entitled (consciously or unconsciously) to present the bill to others or to make them pay.[1] On the other hand, there is such a thing as a constructive duty. Famous are the images of psychoanalyst and infant research pioneer René Spitz. While the baby is being breastfed, he puts his pink in his mother's mouth. Or if he is being fed with a spoon, he will also offer his mum a lick of his treat. Our morality is not only based on an eye for an eye, a tooth for a tooth, but perhaps also on a breast for a breast!

Now, it is normal for us as new-borns to fall into the thick of things. At first, we usually enjoy something extraordinary. We take it for granted that there is a good object out there that will take care of us and suckle us. Donald Winnicott's primary maternal preoccupation[2] and Daniel Stern's motherhood constellation[3] refer to this mother as full of grace. As a mirror and sounding board, she is the archaic mother muse who almost seamlessly attunes to our needs and gestures, creating a fluid *paso doble*.

DOI: 10.4324/9781003394358-14

There is no second chance to make a first impression. The beginning never stops, not even at the end. Thus, in our first period, we usually have an incomparable and unmatched experience by anything that can be found further on (even in the most prosperous life). The seed of our 'True Self' is sown, as is the conviction that we are or can be a Creator.

From a classical Freudian point of view, we inherit the narcissism of our parents. We are His Majesty, the Baby, and in terms of service, our first lackeys remain unsurpassed. They make us feel that everything revolves around us and that a snap of the fingers is enough to fulfil our desires. The inevitable abdication that follows sooner or later is invariably a difficult and laborious process; it never happens without a struggle. Autocracy or aristocracy must make way for law and order, for democracy, a world no longer subordinate to our whim or our will. You can build yourself a throne here and there, with bayonets if necessary. You cannot sit on it (or not as long or comfortably as you want).

Once upon a time, we were supermen, but the real Superman, as he is generally known, was the brainchild of two adolescent Jewish immigrants: Jerry Seigel and Joe Shuster. Jerry lost his father, who was shot in a bank robbery, and Joe's mother was traumatised by Russian pogroms. They were inhibited young men for whom the wishful thinking underlying our muscular superhero was a way of coping with their difficulties.

In their imagination, Superman was born an only child on Krypton and was named Kel-Al. Just before the destruction of his planet, his father, Jor-El, sent him to Earth in a rocket to help and protect humankind. He landed in Millers Field, near Smalltown, Kansas, where he was found by Jonathan and Martha Kent, who had just learned that they could not have children of their own, so they adopted him immediately.

They raised little Clark with high moral standards. They recognised his extraordinary, superhuman powers and talents from an early age. After his parents were killed in a car accident, he left for Metropolis and went to work as a journalist for the Daily Star. Under his somewhat dull office-worker façade, the timid and bespectacled Clark Kent wears his Superman suit. By profession, he is quick to catch up on the latest news. When evil has to be fought, he can change clothes quickly and immediately go out to fight it. While Clark seems invisible to fellow journalist Lois Lane (with whom he is in love), she is completely taken by his alter ego, Superman. He is a God in the depths of her mind.

One of my best friends – balding and overweight like me – recently said he felt like an invisible man. I laughed out loud because it was so recognisable to me. What happened to the days when I felt like Tintin (a journalist like Clark!)[4] with opera singer Bianca Castafiore: my ever-singing mother? Or as a defiantly androgynous David Bowie whom both men and women admired at times? There was a time, much longer ago when I would whizz through space almost every night. Although I kept my arms stretched out against my body, I could steer and accelerate with extreme agility. I could see through walls, and even before Star Trek, I was teleporting.

Kent & I is an anagram of Kinet. Hidden beneath the suit of my invisible Kent is the suit of an I (with the S/the Es) of Superman. Not that I am exceptional in this respect. It is not only poets like Dutch classic Willem Kloos who *hide a God in the depths of their thoughts*.[5] I might refer to Sjoerd Kuyper, Kloos' current compatriot.[6] In one of his poems, he returns to his earliest days when he was able and free to think or imagine himself to be anything he liked: a candle, so he could burn. Or a boy and a girl, kissing each of his hands in turn. If everything went well, we started in such a cradle. Objectively: we were crippled by impotence. Subjectively: we were filled with omnipotence; or with reflections in a Golden I.

Endnotes

1 The balance of giving and receiving is disturbed, which may lead to destructive entitlement, occurring when someone's inherent right or intrinsic entitlement to care is not answered and, as a result, escalates into entitlement. This destructive right entails the risk of scapegoating an innocent third person to balance the account, a phenomenon called the revolving slate (Boszormenyi-Nagy & Spark 1984, p. 66).

2 Winnicott (1956).

3 Stern (1995).

4 *The Adventures of Tintin* is a (comic book) series of twenty-four *bande dessinée* albums created by the Belgian Hergé. The series was one of the most popular comics of the twentieth century. Tintin has been published in more than seventy languages with sales exceeding 200 million copies and has been adapted for radio, television, theatre and film.

5 From a famous poem by the Dutch poet Willem Kloos (2017 [1894]) in which he finds a God in his most intimate thoughts; (with my sincere apologies that the only English page I found is on an astrology website!) see https://www.astro.com/astro-databank/Kloos,_Willem

6 Kuyper (1977).

Chapter 15

Return to Lacan

Mind the Gap

From the outset, I have occasionally commented critically on Solms' neuropsycho-analysis. Still, I often paraphrase a cynical statement by French philosopher Gilles Deleuze from his *Petit Spinoza*: *'Il suffit de ne pas comprendre pour juger'*.[1] To judge something, it suffices not to understand it. Only now that the whole development of Solm's evolving findings and views has been presented does the necessary space for some critical reflections arise.

First of all, I do not call him Mark *Es* without reason.[2] His neuropsychoanalysis is eminently naturalistic and (neuro-) biological. Indeed, it provides a distinction between Id and unconscious, a revision of the drive theory and an update of Freud's *Project*, replacing metapsychological speculations with neuroscientific findings. Solms also develops an exciting view of the dynamic unconscious, but he pays little attention to all its finer points appearing in the clinic, the consulting room and the culture. For all of that, you still have to listen primarily to the many generations (not in the least of clinicians) before him.

To Solms, the Id is a drive system, while the unconscious is a representational, memory or prediction system. The Id is the result of our phylogenetic natural history. Conversely, the unconscious mainly results from our ontogenetic (micro- and macro-) cultural history. In that cultural history, there is, on the one hand, our pre-history. We have no written/declarative sources and must reconstruct what happened based on archaeological finds and (inter-) action patterns. On the other hand, there is history. Here we have text at our disposal, and we constantly try to edit this text into a somewhat coherent story according to an ever-changing perspective. Our historiography is what we have tried to make of our history. We do this consciously or unconsciously, and it is inevitably influenced, more or less, by fears, wishes or fantasies.

In general, Solms' approach sometimes seems a bit too *un*complicated. Everything happens 'naturally' (in the full sense of the word). My reservations, therefore, mainly concern the persistent difficulty of differences between humans and animals. To me, humans do not rank any higher than animals. Every species has assets that others do not have. Much bestiality is also attributed to the 'animal' in

DOI: 10.4324/9781003394358-15

humans. While (industrialised) atrocities like the holocaust (on a large scale) or Marc Dutroux's basement (on a small scale) are paradoxically precisely the privilege of homo sapiens. On the other hand, several ethical (pro-social) values, such as justice and empathy, do not appear to have cultural origins but are equally rooted in our zoological nature.[3]

I mentioned at the start that Solms sometimes devotes (only) one sentence to the imaginary and symbolic (derived as it is from the human corticothalamic mantle). Yet this imaginary and symbolic is what our human life is made of. We are even ready to put this life at stake for unnatural and immaterial goods like God, the homeland, justice, freedom, class struggle, climate matters or our loved ones. Some Things cost a human life. This is known by artists, scientists, politicians and other idealists alike. With a nod to Wilfred Owen's famous poem, this commitment can be far from *Dulce et decorum*.[4]

Furthermore, Solms pays little attention to the fact that humans are fundamentally language-using animals or speaking beings (Lacanian French: *parlêtres*).[5] Chronologically, our pre-history was dominated by action and interaction. '*Am Anfang war die Tat*', according to Freud's famous concluding sentence/Goethe quote of *Totem and taboo*.[6] Initially, the human child cannot speak either (Latin: *in-fans*): the baby *acts*. From birth, there must be an appropriate and specific reaction to our (modern:) *arousal* if a disastrous impact on our psyche is to be avoided. Drive, affect, and trauma are tempered by the imaginary of secure attachment and understood and responded to by the symbolic of law and convention in a context of conferring meaning. It creates a cross-linking that is henceforth found in all human phenomena, that is, all psycho-(patho-)logy.

The body is and remains, however, the infantile in us. It is that which precisely does not (yet) speak. When we are children, our body is disturbing and frightening. The toddler is frightened by the sound of blood pounding in his ear. His parents have to tell him that it is a derivative of the beating of his heart. The physical changes of puberty can be experienced as being as frightening as the Kafkaesque metamorphosis of Gregor Samsa, who has suddenly become an insect. A mediating or remedying intervention of the big Other is also needed. Our feelings are, moreover, physically determined. According to Antonio Damasio's *embodied mind* theory,[7] bodily responses precede feelings logically and chronologically. Over a vertical axis, there is a continuous interaction between bodily sensations and mental functions. Over a horizontal axis, the *infans*, on the other hand, is constantly interacting with the environment/big Other, which, as an ethologically anticipated object, is vital for physical and mental development. The body, a conglomerate of organs, is soothed and calmed down in an interplay of these vertical and horizontal mental functions.

In the most widely read (review) article from *Neuropsychoanalysis,* Aikaterini Fotopoulou and Manos Tsakiris[8] draw on diverse clinical, theoretical and research sources to demonstrate that the physiologically immature and thus vitally dependent human child even needs a 'homeostatically necessary'[9] interaction with this (not anonymous but personal) big Other. This Other sculpts embodied mentalisation, the constitution of a self and the gradual refinement of distinctions between subject and object, self and other and even pleasure and pain. I quote: 'We have made the radical claim that in early infancy when the motor system is immature, proximal interactions are necessary for the active mentalisation of interoceptive states and therefore the corresponding core aspects of the minimal self …' and in continuity with 'the interactive, social self'.[10]

All living beings are not closed but open systems. Indeed, according to Nicola Diamond,[11] our body is primarily a relational body. According to her, not the visual but the tactile of the skin is the semiotic headquarter of our affective and relational life. Presence and absence are registered by our skin rather (or much earlier) than by our eyes. Our skin is also our first home. With Janus's head, it faces the inner and outer world simultaneously. Our Ego is primarily a Skin-Ego ('*Moi-peau*' by Didier Anzieu).[12] It is the product of skin against skin or, in other words, an in-between-skins.[13]

In his 2022 *Intimate Strangers,* Paul Verhaeghe pulls the horizontal axis open even further. The mitochondria in our body contain something other than our DNA. In evolution, they descend from bacteria that got built into our organism and are nestled there. Another body also lives inside our body, too[14] Besides the *world wide web,* there is also Suzanne Simard's *wood wide Web*: under every forest, a network proliferates.[15] According to this view, the world is organised not hierarchically-transcendentally but horizontally-immanently, and sovereignty of the Ego is an illusion because the reality is one of interdependence. As continents we are oceans apart, but on the sea floor we are all connected.

The Language of Animals

Authors as diverse as psychoanalyst Joyce McDougall[16] or infant researchers like Daniel Stern[17] or Robert Emde[18] stress the importance of affective attunement to emotional elements behind the baby's/patient's body language or behaviour. They show that sharing feelings is possible separate from and before verbal language acquisition. Words do not replace this earlier analogical, semiotic or body language but modify and influence it. Very different problems can result from what goes wrong in this process. People may produce words that are not or are insufficiently rooted in a bodily-affective experience. Or conversely, they may be overwhelmed by primitive and disruptive affects they cannot put into words.

Julia Kristeva[19] distinguishes between (dual and pre-Oedipal) semiotic and (triangular and post-Oedipal) symbolic language. In semiotic language, the child produces sounds or babbles in response to the maternal environment. In the so-called *motherese* with which the mother speaks to her child, voice, melody, tone, timbre and, more generally, body language play the leading role. There is a fluidity where the environment and primary process intermingle and overflow. Language is still mainly a matter of imaginary mirroring, where it is not so important *what* but especially *that* and *how* something is said.

Walter Schönau[20] makes a similar distinction between analogue and digital language. Analogue language operates at the level of immediate, intuitive and bodily perception of non-verbal signs that both animals and small children possess. In humans, a digital language superimposes itself onto this, where the relationship between word and meaning becomes arbitrary, based on a symbolic convention. There is no longer a compelling relationship between word and meaning, nor do we ever find the 'right' word again. It will further turn out that Schönau's distinction between analogue and digital language corresponds strongly to Jacques Lacan's imaginary and symbolic order. At the beginning of his teaching, the ethological or the imaginary was central. We have them in common with the animals. They, too, understand the language of attachment and seduction, of taking cover, of dominance and submission within a particular pecking order. It determines intercourse between conspecifics where all kinds of *size* do *matter.* Think of the nightingale's song or the peacock's tail flaunting as evolutionarily escalated image-building. For their respective survival, the benefit of these gadgets is debatable. But in terms of procreative success, they are of significant benefit. Therefore, what is suitable for the species does not always work beneficially for the individual!

Eduardo Kohn[21] wrote a wonderful book about how the jungle thinks and how people in this jungle think. Philosopher and semiotician Charles Peirce strongly inspire his descriptions.[22] The latter's tripartite division between icon, index and symbol may be sufficiently familiar. At the icon's heart is the similarity of the image (including the sound image): a particular visual pattern or onomatopoeia whose *Gestalt* refers directly to something else. The index is a trace: smoke relates to fire, a broken branch to a passer-by. All the jungle and all the living things inhabiting it participate in both these signs. It is only the symbol that is based on convention. Its importance, according to Kohn, is overstated just because it is uniquely human!

Especially in Jacques Lacan's oeuvre, the distinction between humans and other animals is a constant. Animal psychology is entirely defined by the imaginary, while the added dimension of the symbolic complicates human psychology. The paternal function of the symbolic order underlies the regulation of kinship relations and hence the gap between humans and animals. Yet he states – to all intents and purposes – in his *Ecrits* that 'the doctrine of a discontinuity between animal psychology and human psychology is far away from our thought'.[23] Still, the entry into symbolic language and its law and order *does* make a difference. After all, it exemplifies a broader symbolic order of laws and rules it establishes and underpins. The symbolic order is that of signifiers by which we name the world and assign ourselves a place about who or what surrounds us. It provides an order based not on resemblance (as in the imaginary) but on difference.[24] Difference between man and woman, girl and mother, man and animal. I referred earlier to Schönau with the distinction between analogue and digital language.[25] The former is based on similarity (the grooves in the gramophone record and the waves of sound), the latter on a (mere) binary arrangement that can (re-)write the world in endless ways. After all, simplicity and complexity are not mutually exclusive. I said it before: a CD may consist of an astronomical collection of simple ones and zeros, but simultaneously it sounds like a Cantata by Bach.

Our typically human capacity for symbolic language serves roughly four functions.[26] It contributes to identity acquisition (I am the son of, a friend of, work at, and live there). It contributes to cognitive and emotional communication; it is necessary for self-awareness. Last but not least, it gradually contributes to the increasing mastery of drive, affect and trauma. Language development occurs in a *joint (ad)venture* with the big Other (usually the mother), on the model of which other social ties/relationships will form later. Lacan's maxim that the unconscious is the discourse of the Other[27] implies that the unconscious is not the archaic and primordial realm of drives and instincts but the domain of (micro- or macro-) cultural and symbolic constructs that exert their determining influence outside or without our awareness.

Grand Canyon

Language develops gradually and chronologically for most post-Freudians. It is an (evolutionary) biological model of crops that slowly mature. This is explicitly *not* Lacan's view.[28] To him, moreover, the human condition is *structurally* characterised by a particular type of response (neurotic, perverse or psychotic) to a lack of being that symbolic language logically causes.[29] Man ultimately has a gap to close. In this context, Paul Verhaeghe refers to the warning heard all over the London Underground: *Mind the gap, mind the gap, mind the gap.*[30]

Undoubtedly, this immediately indicates the enormous chasm[31] emerging within the psychoanalytic world. Feel free to call it a *Grand Canyon* Jacques Lacan has opened up by giving Freud's ideas a linguistic[32] turn. Over-adaptationist psychoanalysis is disrupted and lifted from its hinges at a stroke. Indeed, the entry into language and symbolic order, according to him, creates an unbridgeable gap between nature and culture. The original immediacy (of the animal in its habitat/biotope) is lost in the process. While language is our home, it can also feel like a prison from which we try to escape (in all possible and impossible ways). Man creates a world and has (or *is*) an inherently unfulfillable and inappropriate desire. This desire is linked, after all (not to an object but) to the *lack of* an object.[33] To Lacan, paradoxically, it is *the* object of psychoanalysis even.[34]

According to Lacanian psychoanalysis, man also owes three lost and longed-for objects to symbolic language. These are the Thing, the small object a, and the phallus, around which his psychosexual and sociocultural desires pivot.[35] They belong to the Real, the Imaginary and the Symbolic, respectively. The Thing and object small a refer to pre-Oedipal lacks. They are, as it were, relics of the early mother-child fusion we nostalgically yearn for or which cause our desire, precisely by their loss.[36] In a Lacanian view, desire is caused by loss, whereas to him loss is, in turn, the object of the drive. The drive circles repetitively around an unattainable object, and this repetition produces *jouissance*/enjoyment. Desire puts a stop to this *jouissance.* Desire limits *jouissance;* in this sense, it is a defence against the death drive. The drive keeps missing the object. Although counterintuitive (because unconscious), what we do *not* want gives us enjoyment. Paradoxically, we enjoy *not* getting what we want. With a nod to Panksepp and Berridge, we enjoy seeking (and not finding) what we want.

The phallus refers to an Oedipal lack in a (not dual but) triangular relationship.[37] Freud introduced it as a third term with a significant signifying role. The absolute primacy of the phallus has even become a doctrinal, if not dogmatic, basis of Lacanian theory. It is the signifier of signifiers, the privileged signifier. It symbolises that we can never have enough or be enough to be *the One and Only* to the big Other and thus fully satisfy the desire of this big Other. It is far beyond our scope to elaborate fully on all this here and now. It has been covered in some of my previous publications,[38] and as the best warm-up, I gladly recommend Lionel Bailly's *Lacan for Beginners.*[39]

Essentially human to Lacan are not harmony but rupture, the gap and division. *The* law of man is the law of language.[40] Language and symbolic order are external and pre-existent and constitute the unnatural nature of man as a speaking being. To Lacan, a psychoanalysis focused on adaptation ignores the alienating implications of the Ego (for him to be understood as imaginary, specular, a mirage or mirror). This kind of psychoanalysis also has a naïve conception of reality (which, after all, as the real, is never knowable and perceivable as such).[41] Development is not a merely natural (that is, in this context (neuro-) biological) process, but something that is motorised by (the desire of) the Other. Ariane Bazan repeatedly speaks of physical pushing and social pulling in this context. Nor is it a linear process in time, but it is characterised by posteriority. History is constantly being written and rewritten, and even the (typically human) future perfect tense (what will be told about me at my funeral?) affects today. Development is not a fluidity of gradual transitions but is characterised by leaps/choices by which the subject[42] manifests itself.[43]

Man is governed not so much by instincts (as fixed and innate relations to the object) but by drives and cultural complexes. The ultimate way the drive constellation organises itself has always and inevitably been something of a bricolage.[44] There is no ultimate synthesis or normality that would result from a natural developmental process, as, for example, 'mature, genital love'.[45] There is only an always intimate relationship that each subject assumes towards an object small a, that he considers (in an imaginary way) to be his Thing.[46] It follows that psychoanalysis has nothing to gain from biological or psychological developments reducing it unnecessarily to an ideology of adaptation. Indeed, between man and the world, there is an unbridgeable gap.[47]

Jacques Lacan distinguishes between three registers that structure the human condition. There is the specifically human, symbolic order of language and lack, signifier and difference, law and the No or the Name of the Father[48] (in French, *Non* and *Nom* are homophonic). Neurally (and speculatively), they could be situated neocortically. There is the imaginary order of body image and mirroring, supposed wholeness, appearance and seduction. Neurally, they could be located in the limbic system. Finally, there is the order of the real as the neither imaginary nor symbolically (quite) imaginable remainder: the noumenal (and deeply subcortical) of Thing, drive or trauma. In Lacan's thinking, this real (albeit as an inconceivable category) receives a proper place. The real is (as in the dream or the drive-root of the symptom) even the navel/mycelium around which all imaginary-symbolic spins gravitate.[49] It is also the famous grain of sand around which the mother(-of-pearl) forms its more or less shiny layers.[50] This real is colonised but never (completely) conquered by ever-advancing science. This is true of the outer world, where Star Trek's *final frontier* is never within our reach, neither in the Big Bang's ultra-large nor the Higgs boson's ultra-small. But this is equally true of our inner world. According to neuroscientist V.S. Ramachandran, we know as many possible brain states as there are elementary particles in the universe. In this sense, our head is as infinite as the macrocosm.[51] But to all intents and purposes, this impossibility does not negate the value or importance of a scientific vocation or activity. Indeed, Freud firmly replied to those who opposed science: as if we could build bridges out of cardboard![52]

The Big Other

Earlier I referred repeatedly to a famous Lacanian maxim: *L'inconscient, c'est le discours de l'Autre.* The unconscious is the discourse of the big Other. What is meant is the symbolic order as the body of laws, norms, rules, social codes and social institutions, and – above all: language. This big Other should be distinct from a concrete person who, on the other hand, does represent or embody this symbolic order. Through parents, a child acquires the language and the laws, rules and social codes of the group to which he belongs and thus receives an identity. Since we always belong to multiple groups – family, work, the country we live in – we always carry multiple identities with us as well. Identity is thus embedded in history – in your family story, the language you speak, and the stories that have left their mark. Through that symbolic order, we acquire identity and the capacity to handle the drive or affect regulation. Indeed, through the language we are given, we learn to name all kinds of fragmented and indeterminate sensations ('affects'). They become 'feelings' we can then place in a narrative and thus connect to events and people in the present and the past.

The identity gained through the symbolic order is opposed to the idea of identity as a supposed unity. Lacan, after all, opposed the idea that there is such a thing as an authentic, unadulterated and unique Self hidden deep within us. He talks about an 'imaginary position' in this context. He refers to the moment when the mother holds a small child in front of the mirror and says: 'Look, that's you'. This self-image as a total image is an imaginary *mirage* because the child still experiences himself as completely fragmented and, above all, powerless. Moreover, this self-image comes from outside: the mother (or her eyes) holds up the mirror image. According to Lacan, this imaginary position is one of fictitious omnipotence. It leads us into a 'dual relationship', in which one is the mirror of the

other, a relationship that, apart from omnipotence and wholeness, is also characterised by envy, rivalry and competition (things that are in no way conceptualised
within attachment theory).

Returning to the etymology, the word 'identity' refers to the Latin *identitas,*
meaning 'equality' or 'the same'. In this way, identity does not refer to a unique
hidden self but rather to the micro- and macro-culture of which you are a part
and with which you have identified or from which you have distanced/separated
yourself. According to Lacan, the initial mirroring relationship can only be broken
through the symbolic order. This introduces lack, imperfection and boundaries.
Not only are we 'influenced' by the (structure) of this language, but we are also
dependent on it. We are, for this reason, not creatures of nature but creatures of
culture. According to Lacan, we fail as biological beings[53]: we can hardly fall back
on natural behaviour patterns from birth. We rely on external guidance. And this
comes from culture, which helps compensate for the biological deficit. Where the
animal is attuned to its environment, humans are much less so. Man is alienated
from his environment and broken open, as it were.

Jacques Lacan also makes a distinction (to some extent parallel to the real, the
imaginary and the symbolic) between need, demand and desire. The need is a
purely biological given. It springs from the organism, and its satisfaction immediately (but often also temporarily) silences this need. Born in helpless dependence,
the human child cannot satisfy its needs and must use its vocal cords. The need
must be articulated to become a question to the big Other. The presence of this big
Other becomes a requirement in itself, and it goes beyond mere need satisfaction
because this presence comes to symbolise love on behalf of this big Other. The
demand gradually acquires a double function: (1) it articulates a need, and (2) it
becomes a demand for love. The big Other, in turn, may fulfil the need, but the hunger for love is never (ultimately) satisfied. Even when the child has what it needs,
there remains an unfulfilled demand for love, and longing/desire is this inevitable
residual. In common parlance: it is never *that,* and it is never enough.

Needs are biologically compelling: without food, drink, air, sleep, proper
body temperature and so on, not only does our homeostasis perish, but we die.
We can neither sublimate nor symbolise these needs. They need to be satisfied
energetically-materially. The demand for love is of an entirely different, immaterial order. The mother's breast is, therefore, the place where hunger and desire
meet. We may be able to survive without love, but whether we can call that *to
feel alive* is very much the question.[54] For example, we can feed someone with a
feeding tube. The need for nutrients (Solms constantly talks about *needs*) is satisfied. But we could also provide the same hungry person with his favourite dish
(whether or not lovingly prepared).

In fancy terms, psychoanalysis is not about survival but about feeling and
being alive in a more existential-affective way.[55] Even if all our material *needs* are
satisfied, we can still be miserable. When asked what is at stake when we have
missed an encounter with happiness, the philosopher might answer: wisdom, but

the psychoanalyst would possibly answer: desire or lack. This desire/lack is problematic but necessary. Love helps (not to fill but) to mind this gap. On the other hand, all attempts to deny the gap are fatal to us as subjects. After all, the gap is constitutive of having or being a desire. To Lacanians, this desire resides in the gap between the need and the demand for love.[56] It directs itself pre-eminently towards all those symbolic-imaginary goods and values at the heart of our happiness and spiritual life.[57]

Endnotes

1 Deleuze (2003, p. 33). More generally, judgements are often made about anything and everything. This not hindered by sufficient knowledge or understanding.
2 Playing with semantics and phonemes, I call Mark S Mark Es. Among close friends, I myself sometimes sign (only because of my 'haircut') as Mark Skinhead (or as Dr Ive).
3 This is often emphasised by primatologist Frans de Waal see, for example, 2017. In his Yale lab, Paul Bloom (2013) also convincingly demonstrates how the evolutionary component of good and evil can already be established in babies; obviously, taking good care of one's offspring and family provides an adaptive advantage and holds true when extended to larger groups.
4 I am of course referring to Wilfred Owen's concluding verses after a First World War gas attack (Owen 1917). See https://en.wikisource.org/wiki/Poems_by_Wilfred_Owen/ Dulce_et_Decorum_est
5 In this context, I will immediately quote Lacan from his Seminar XI on 15/04/1964 (1998, p. 126): 'I will ask analysts a straight question: *have you ever, for a single moment, the feeling that you are handling the clay of instinct?* [...] The unconscious is the sum of the effects of speech on a subject, at the level at which the subject constitutes himself out of the effects of the signifier'.
6 Freud (1912–1913a, b).
7 Damasio (1994).
8 Fotopoulou and Tsakiris (2017).
9 Ibid., p. 2.
10 Ibid., p. 22.
11 Diamond (2013).
12 Anzieu (1985).
13 Thys (2015a).
14 Verhaeghe (2022, p. 56).
15 Ibid., p. 61.
16 McDougall (1982).
17 Stern (1985).
18 Emde (1991).
19 Kristeva (1984).
20 Schönau (2002).
21 Kohn (2013).
22 Charles Sander Peirce (1839–1914) see (1994).
23 Lacan (1966, p. 484).
24 Lacan (1957).
25 Bateson (2002 [1979]): *a bit is a bit that makes a difference.*
26 Verhaeghe (2002, p. 148).
27 Lacan (1966). One can find in the unconscious the effects of speech on the subject i.e. the unconscious is the effect of the signifier on the subject.

28 Declercq (2000, p. 85ff).
29 Verhaeghe (2002, p. 170).
30 Verhaeghe (2001, p. 8).
31 To Lacan, there is a gap in man. After all, he is not one but two with nature. This is, in the first instance, and as a consequence of, mirror self-cognition/the mirror stage, when man identifies himself with his (mirror) image in a leap forward and at the same time misses an underlying and alienating field of tension. Indeed, through deception, the imaginary precisely covers this gap. It covers the inner divisions and presents us with an imagined or imaginary sense of unity and wholeness. In an allusion to *hominisation*, however, there remains a missing link. Man is inevitably on horseback on or trapped in the gap between nature and culture. His impossible task is 'to mind the gap '. In a Nietzschean paraphrase, he stretches a tightrope above this abyss. Fundamental disharmony is inescapably man's fate. Any human science worthy of the name moves between explaining and understanding, natural sciences and hermeneutics (Luyten, Blatt & Corveleyn 2006). It is an uncomfortable but inevitable split without which human truth is violated (Nieweg 2005).
32 Jacques Lacan gives his linguistic interpretation with his neologism *linguistery* (English: *linguistrickery*): contraction of linguistics and hysteria or a hysterical transformation of linguistics. For details, see Milner (2000)
33 '*l'objet de la psychanalyse est le manque d'un objet*' (1953, p. 268). The object of psychoanalysis is the lack of an object (my translation).
34 Lacan (1966b, p. 12).
35 For further elaboration, see, for example, Kinet (2018)
36 The Thing and object small a are elaborated by Lacan in Seminar VII and VIII, respectively. Das Ding/the Thing is the object of desire. It is a lost object continually looked for, the unforgettable and forbidden object of incestuous desire. It appears as the Supreme Good, but to attain it the subject must go beyond the pleasure principle and the enjoyment into the unenjoyable and causes suffering or evil (cf *le Mal* in Charles Baudelaire's *Les Fleurs du Mal*).
37 For current views on the Oedipus complex, see Kinet and Heuves (2019). In his IV Seminar (1956–1957) Lacan elaborates on the phallus. In the distinction between phallus and penis, the first refers to an imaginary object. This imaginary phallus is perceived by the child as THE object of the mother's desire so the child seeks to identify with this object and attempts to be the imaginary phallus. In order to assume castration the child must renounce the possibility of being this phallus. The symbolic phallus comes to be the signifier of the Other's desire and the signifier of *jouissance*/enjoyment. The law of the father/ *la fonction paternelle* introduces the phallus as a third and imaginary term. The Oedipus complex is thus quadrangular. In short: three Oedipal stages constitute the subject. 1. The paternal function inaugurates the primacy given to the phallus by culture. 2. The father intervenes as the one who forbids the child access to the mother. The child is *not* her phallic object. 3. The child is liberated and deprived of the (incestuous) object of desire, and wanting to *be* the phallus changes into having (or not having) the phallus.
38 Kinet (2017).
39 Bailly (2009). Lacan de-literalises Freudian concepts and he 'liberates' psychoanalysis from biologism. De-literalises: the literal penis is replaced by the symbolic penis or phallus. Castration anxiety and penis envy are not determined by anatomy. The possible loss of everything having phallic significance for a woman (her hair, breasts, looks etc) can cause castration anxiety, and men can also be envious of the success, money, and women of others. Away from biologism: there is a difference between organic needs we have in common with animals and desire arising from an inner sense of lack or absence. The – Lacanian – phallus is an empty signifier. In a somewhat bold metaphor, it is an invisible nail from which hangs an empty frame on a wall that does not exist. It is highly

significant and at the same time *an sich* meaningless. In one context, a Ferrari counts as phallic; in another, a Morris Mini, a library or a football jersey. Unlike biological sex or psychological gender, Lacanian sexuality revolves around the subjective relationship to the phallus. Male: around the desire to have the phallus. Female: (also) around the desire to be the enigmatic phallus. Man's enjoyment is phallic; woman's enjoyment (also) goes beyond this boundary. We desire to be or to have the object of the other's desire. To have or to be what the other lacks. By definition, what the other desires or lacks is the phallus. See a later note.

40 Lacan (1966b, p. 272).

41 Alienation, to Lacan, is constitutive of the human subject, who is divided in a fundamental and unresolvable way. We can never feel whole, complete or coherent. This is due to the identification with a literal or figurative mirror image that underlies our self(-image). This is a consequence of the mirror stage, which is, on the one hand, a developmental stage, but on the other hand, a (cf. the Kleinian) position that for the rest of life characterises the relationship to self and other. The alienation is captured pointedly in Arthur Rimbaud's verse: *Je est un autre*. 'I is another'. Alienation is inherent to the order of the imaginary, which finds its most essential expression in it. The sixteenth chapter of Lacan's Seminar XI (1973 p 185-195) is devoted to alienation and its related separation.

42 In Lacan's thought the term 'subject' has a specific meaning. At first, it was meant a 'human being' (1966a, p 75), then it meant the analysand (ibid., p. 83). Still, there is the personal subject, whose uniqueness is constituted by self-affirmation (ibid. p 207-8). The subject is not simply equivalent to a conscious sense of agency (the Ego as an imaginary illusion) but to the unconscious; Lacan's 'subject' is the subject of the unconscious. It is *'le sujet de l'énonciation'* (and not *'de l'énoncé'*): The subject of speaking, not the subject of the spoken. In his *mathèmes* the subject is represented with the symbol S: a homophone of Freud's term Es.

43 A reference to Jean-Paul Sartre (1996 [1946], Sartre certainly inspired Lacan but is hardly mentioned by him) is appropriate here. *L'existence précède l'essence* is *the* point of *L'existentialisme est un humanisme*. The animal is *plein d'être*, it lives according to its (natural) essence. Man has the freedom to evade his nature. He can invent (including himself). In Hannah Arendt's terms, he is capable of 'natality' (1998 [1958]).

44 Safouan (2005, pp. 57–59).

45 Van Haute (2000, p. 140).

46 Kinet (2002, 2017).

47 Van Haute (2000, pp. 25–26).

48 In the Lacanian theory of psychosis (elaborated especially in his Seminar III (1955-1956)), the Name of the Father is foreclosed (*Verwerfung*). Two conditions are required for psychosis to emerge: inheritance and foreclosure resulting in the most notable language phenomena in psychosis.

49 Freud (1900a, p. 573, 1900b, p. 609).

50 Freud (1905a, p. 112).

51 Cf the interlude 'Infinitely Less than Zero' where reference is made to Matte-Blanco's (1988) *The unconscious as infinite sets.*

52 Freud (1933a, p. 227, 1933b, p. 177). I quote in full Freud's answer *avant-la-lettre* to the excesses of a culture of opinion. The postmodernist *anything goes*: 'If it did not matter what we think, if there were no knowledge that stands out among our opinions because of its conformity to reality, we would be allowed to build bridges of cardboard as well as of stone, to inject the patient with a decigram instead of a centigram of morphine, to use tear gas instead of ether for anaesthesia. Even intellectual anarchists, however, would vigorously reject these practical applications of their theory'. Cf: Prayers can bring us to heaven, not to the moon.

53 There is something inadequate about human biology, a 'vital insufficiency' *(insuffisance vitale)* (Lacan 1949c, p. 90).

54 Indeed, it *may be* survival because didn't René Spitz's (1945) research on hospitalism clearly show a *failure to thrive* (aka growth retardation) in children who received insufficient emotional nourishment from their parents?

55 Regarding this existential component I might refer for example to the existential psychotherapy of Irvin Yalom (1980). He elaborates on some of the most important problematic givens of the human condition: isolation, responsibility, meaninglessness, mortality and freedom. He adds one more level/dimension to Maslow's pyramid: not self-realisation but self-transcendence. In short: one comprehends oneself in order not to be preoccupied with oneself (ibid., p. 439). Solms would probably argue that these 'existential' concerns can to some extent be correlated to their emotional-instinctive counterparts like separation, care or fear.

56 In short: demand minus need = desire. In an example from everyday life: you can feed the hungry who ask for food. In that case, you respond to the demand and satisfy the need. But you can also prepare a mushroom risotto for a friend invited to dinner. The friend asked is not hungry, but he *desires* to come for a visit, and the dinner is centred around appetite and enjoyment. Another example: you don't give the birthday boy/girl a present he/she needs but something he/she enjoys. What kind of husband would provide a flatiron for a gift?

57 For example, in consumer-capitalist enjoyment we can get all kinds of satisfaction. Still, they don't lead to happiness but to a sort of depressive *hedonia* (Fisher 2009: the inability to do anything else except pursue pleasure. Something is missing – feeling without the awareness that this mysterious, missing enjoyment lies *beyond* the pleasure principle). Paradoxically we can feel all the more miserable. We have got to 'savour' the lack of the missing object or of missing the object. In fact, we are surrounded by a huge number of objects, but only those objects that are scarce, unavailable or unattainable are attractive or seductive. The lack of an object produces some kind of divine spark and this lack keeps us going. Vincent Hanna/Al Pacino in Michael Mann's motion picture *Heat*: 'All I am is what I am (I would say: keep) going after'.

Chapter 16

Interlude

Manneken Pis

Most major cities have sky-scraping phallic symbols. The Eiffel Tower in Paris, the former World Trade Centre towers in New York and the Burj Khalifa in Dubai consecutively surpassed each other. Brussels lags somewhat behind in this regard. Our capital has only the balls of the Atomium and the penis of *Manneken Pis* to offer. Typically Belgian, our little hero does not take the biscuit but makes fun of power. For example, he makes silly fools of the Goliaths of this world. In a sense, it is Andy Warhol's *avant-la-lettre*: Art is what you can get away with.

In the fall of 2020, three well-known Flemish men from the show(!)business made headlines because their nude images circulated on social media. They had been seduced by a lady into posting dick pics. Nowadays, in the context of sexting, it is pretty standard for young people to photograph their intimate parts and distribute them to potential suitors. However, the fact that three adult men (officially engaged in a close relationship and the public eye) were tempted to do this was unknown and caused quite a stir. It gave rise to a lot of consternation and hilarity. The partner of one of these men now lives elsewhere. The fate of the other relationships remains private for the time being.

There is, of course, a phase in our development in which the phallus plays a leading role, according to Freud. If I am to believe my aunt (she is the only witness living today), I, for example, was very proud when I was allowed to pull out my specimen and pee standing against a tree as a toddler. That, here and there, a woman is envious of us for this male accomplishment may be evident from, among other things, the invention of the pee funnel. Moreover, when the phallus appears on the scene in an erect state, it quickly acquires symbolic significance. Since the agricultural revolution and the associated patriarchy, it has replaced the Venus of Willendorf as a fertility symbol. More generally, it represents power and authority within the symbolic-imaginary order. The female then degenerated into a kind of land ownership. In more poetic terms: her womb is a field where males and females root for some eternity.

Let me make a jump to the clinic. Hilde is in weekly psychotherapy. She suffered greatly from her *Godfather*-like father. Dominant and transgressive, he was a kind of *Darth Vader*.[1] Out of fear and a need for love, she has always been very obliging

DOI: 10.4324/9781003394358-16

and almost religiously devoted to him. Although he died years ago, she has not yet been able to entirely cast off the yoke of his 'super' Ego.

In the first of two consecutive sessions, Hilde talks about her husband, Robert. He is – not coincidentally – the antithesis of her father and, despite his age, retains something childlike and affectionate. She watches television while their dog Boris rests his head on her lap. She loves stroking Boris, and it is with some disbelief that she notices that Robert sometimes seems genuinely jealous of their four-legged friend. When Boris leaves his luxurious position, Robert takes up the vacant place and claims the same affectionate and cherished treatment. This annoys Hilde, but mostly she feels some pity.

In the next session, she relates that her husband suddenly dropped his pants the previous Sunday afternoon in the living room. He had shaved off his pubic hair and asked her what she thought. Hilde was bewildered and speechless. Immediately, she prepared to let him have his way that evening. Only then could she relax again for a few months. 'Men have their needs, of course'.

After previous descriptions of her partner, I am somewhat surprised by Robert's sudden and unexpected démarche. At first, I think of her father. He often commented on her bosom and had once touched her breasts, too: an aspect of him she could not process. Did Robert's exhibition trigger old traumas? I invite her to speak her mind.

She takes a very different tack. For example, she tells me that Patrick, their only son, now growing taller than Robert, had mentioned just days before that he was beginning to get hair in his armpits. He found this gross and planned to shave it off. Could it be that her husband was jealous of Boris and their son? That he wanted to regress to pre-puberty? I had heard before that some women would position themselves naked in front of the TV to attract their husband's interest. But this manoeuvre?

Of course, the fact that Robert shaved off his pubic hair may be understood in the context of today's pornification, which involves imitating the bodies and acts that reign supreme. I knew he was a particularly ardent viewer of nature documentaries and political talk shows. Not that one precludes the other, of course. Hilde found his performance mostly awkward, if not clumsy. Although she was shocked, she felt more pity than fear or disgust.

In this context, another line of thinking is more likely. Robert wants precisely to return to a pre-pubescent state to regain the attention and fondness of his wife. By defacing himself, he thinks he is or has 'It' for Hilde and tries to capture her attention, if not to monopolise her.

According to Michel Thys,[2] Wilfred Bion's container-contained model caused a paradigmatic shift within psychoanalysis. Classic psychoanalytic concepts such as resistance, inner conflict, infantile sexuality, dream labour or the Oedipus complex have all become somewhat repressed. So what are we to do with Hilde, Robert and Patrick (for Boris, presumably, it makes no difference)? In a Lacanian view,[3] the Oedipus complex exhibits not a triangular but a quadrangular structure: father, mother, child and phallus. The latter is supposed to satisfy the mother's desire (entirely). It can appear in a thousand guises or fragments. Paraphrasing Freud, you can only pay in the country's currency you enter. In right-wing circles, a Porsche counts as phallic. In left-wing circles, a rickety two h.p., and with the Greens, an electric bike is probably the best way to 'score'.

The phallus, like money, makes the world go round, but it can be found neither at the airport lost property desk nor at Wilfred Bion's counter. All 'semblance', it only *seems* and is made of absence. It is a hidden and gilded emptiness.

Endnotes

1 Darth Vader is considered to be one of the biggest baddies in Western film culture. After the release of Star Wars' *The Empire Strikes Back*, director George Lucas stated that the name Vader was based upon the German/Dutch-language word *Vater* or *vader*, making the named representative of a 'Dark Father' see https://www.forbes.com/sites/quora/2017/11/28/did-german-speakers-understand-the-darth-vader-reveal-before-anyone-else/?sh=6c677306605e
2 Thys (2015b, p. 88).
3 Lacan (1994, pp. 240–241).

Chapter 17

Driven Signifiers

Phantom Pain

From the start, I have referred to Bazan as a figurehead of Lacanian neuropsychoanalysis. She obtained a PhD in biology and psychology, and through her neuroscience research with Howard Shevrin, she evolved toward neuropsychoanalysis.[1] Bazan recently made the Lacanian contribution to the revisited *Clinical Studies*[2] and is preparing a book entitled *Lacanian Neuropsychoanalysis*. Following Mark Solms' biological and physical excursions, her approach, as will be seen, is more in line with Nietzsche's[3] *allzumenschliches* as it appears in the consulting room.

Adolf Grünbaum's scientific requirement was that empirical evidence of psychoanalytic assumptions should also be provided independently of their clinical setting/methodology. Well, the methods of Shevrin's lab succeeded in demonstrating a neuro-inhibition that can most simply be understood as an unconscious defence. Using subliminal stimuli (in the context of *priming*)[4] and evoked potentials, they found independent, non-behavioural and objective indications at the brain level that clinical interpretations made a priori by psychoanalysts could also be confirmed independently (i.e. theory-independent). As a brain phenomenon, Alpha synchronisation appears to be the physiological counterpart of unconscious defence mechanisms.[5] They target affectively charged words/signifiers, and they have an internal origin. Shevrin's results could only be understood as expressing a complex and dynamic unconscious due to early childhood conflicts around 'scandalous' themes.

Furthermore, her chapter in our book was entitled *Signifiers in Brain Tissue*. As early as 1953, Lacan had proposed that Freud's ideas on the functioning of the unconscious (and mental life in general) should be understood within the context of linguistic theory. In his view, the unconscious comprises signifiers, the most elementary language units. Like de Saussure,[6] Lacan distinguishes signifier from signified. The signified concerns the concept or the idea that the linguistic sign conveys, while the signifier only refers to the acoustic image that makes up the sign.[7] In the processes of speech or writing, signifiers are related to signifieds, which results in the creation of signification.[8] Ferdinand de Saussure asserted the predominance of the signified over the signifier. This implies that language is used

DOI: 10.4324/9781003394358-17

to transfer and express meaning. Lacan,[9] however, clearly argues for the opposite by considering the signifier as primordial. At the level of the unconscious, it is the signifier that predominates, and it is the signifier that establishes the logic of how symptoms are organised.

Indeed, this typically Lacanian emphasis on the signifier was already present in Bazan's first and original neuropsychoanalysis of what she calls a phantom.[10] I will briefly outline her view on this. When you get started on something, explicitly or implicitly, 'it' feels good as long as you get 'there'. After all, the brain has two feedback systems to monitor movement. The somatosensory cortex calculates where you will end up, and the proprioceptive system links back to whether the intended goal was achieved. The latter is called the 'efferent copy'. If both systems agree, everything 'fits'. However, an incongruity arises between intention and behaviour if you do not achieve the intended goal. A (merely '*phantomatic*') intention then does not get confirmation from the proprioceptive system, triggering anxiety and discomfort. Compare it to descending a staircase and suddenly discovering a missing step (although one more was expected). In Solms' terms, an unpleasant surprise awaits you. The energy bound under the form of a prediction becomes dissolved and produces anxiety.

In Bazan's Lacanian view, the unconscious consists of signifiers and is linguistically structured following Lacan. These signifiers, moreover, have materiality. They are phonemic but also motoric because they are articulated or written (even internally/when silent). According to Bazan, actions and unarticulated/unwritten/unspoken words produce phantoms. To illustrate this, in her book, she uses the coercive phantoms of the *Rat Man*[11] to demonstrate multiple false entanglements of signifiers. His associative signifier chain shifts from the intention to marry his lover ('*heiraten*') to other signifiers in which the phoneme '*rat*' recurs: *Frau Hofrat* (the governess with whom he played sexual games), the fear of *rats* or the German '*Raten*', referring to debit accounts. Words and ideas that were repressed turn out to cause phantoms. They fail to discharge and cause anxiety. The automaton does not work. The Rat Man's symptoms are understood to result from an essentially linguistic unconscious playing with signifiers, which occurs unknowingly and demonically. Regardless of their semantics, signifiers haunt our psyche, they are carriers of affect, and their meaning can only be elucidated in the correct context.[12] I would like, in this connection, to paraphrase Jacques Derrida.[13] His famous '*il n'y a pas de hors texte*' then becomes '*il n'y a pas de hors* con-*texte*'.

Apple

Not just to Bazan[14] but to all Lacanians, the human condition is fundamentally related to the ability to wield a symbolic language.[15] Signifiers are constituent elements. The interpretation of phonemes depends entirely on the surrounding phonemes. This context-dependence of phonemes (I repeat: considered as phonetically or sensorimotor expressible objects) is un-natural. In nature, objects retain their meaning regardless of context. An apple remains an apple.[16] Whether hanging from a tree, lying on the ground or rolling down a slope. Its analogous stability of meaning is, after all, evolutionarily significant. All animal candidates can thus quickly find their way to the apple without it presenting them with complicated epistemological or linguistic issues. We can refer to Jean-Paul Sartre's existentialist views for this anthropological difference.[17] To him, the animal is (full of) being: *plein d'être.* Its essence entirely defines it. Man, by contrast, is *néant:* a nothing. Paraphrasing British philosopher John Gray: *humans are the void looking at itself.*[18] Their existence precedes their essence. They always possess the (staggering) freedom to withdraw from nature or *their* nature. Hannah Arendt[19] calls this the specifically human natality: his extraordinary ability always to start entirely afresh.

But I will continue concerning the signifier. In humans, to one subject, the word 'apple' is linked to Adam and Eve and the Garden of Eden, and another, to the apple of discord – underlying the Trojan War. It can evoke associations with the apple that Wilhelm Tell managed to hit with a bow and arrow or with the orchard at Woolsthorpe Manor, where Isaac Newton saw (with all its consequences) an apple fall and so on. Moreover, to most of us, the word 'apple' is associated with the Apple computer and (at least, as a written word) with an appeal (to others for help).[20] In each case, the context determines the meaning and scope of the word 'apple' for the person involved. Man is eminently capable of suspending his interpretation of the word 'apple' to consider the surrounding signifiers. He owes this ability to an exceptionally elaborate circuit of inhibition. It is located behind his high forehead: the prefrontal cortex. Translated into everyday language, words are continuously stripped of their ambiguity. For instance, in poetry, (verbal) humour and other word games, this ambiguity can come into its own again with all the (more or less forbidden) *fun* that this implies.[21]

The peculiarity of signifiers described, the symbolic order, creates a gap. With Lacan, this gap appears in many variations of the theme. There is the world-famous painting *La trahison des images* alias *Ceci n'est pas une pipe* by the Belgian surrealist painter René Magritte. There is always a gap between the Thing and the image or word we attach to it. It is the famous Kantian caesura between *noumenon* and *phenomenon*, where immediacy is lost. It determines the human lack of being. After Lacan, I have already called it his *manque-à-être*[22] or his want-to-be.[23] *Ceci n'est pas une pipe.* The Thing (*an sich*) is thus simultaneously killed and born.[24] In this way, another rupture occurs, with man losing a piece (of himself, too). In a Lacanian view, object small a is an imaginary remainder of this loss and functions as an object-cause of desire. For example, in romantic love: in the eyes of the lover, the beloved has *something* that arouses desire. It cannot be put into words, but it *drives* lovers towards some form of 'healing' and a supposedly-original but mythical enjoyment. This movement has something transgressive (Freud[25]: 'It takes an obstacle to propel the libido upwards'), which can also be harmful (if not deadly).[26] I will return to this later on.

The gap, on the other hand, is also constitutive of the subject itself.[27] Lacan saw a man (as Freud did before him) as biologically immature and incomplete. He has a fragmented body consisting of still disorganised *partial* drives seeking healing/wholeness in the mirage of the mirror image. In an alienating movement, we identify with this, as described in his famous (and essentially narcissistic and imaginary) mirror stage.[28] Also, purely somatically, many gaps occur. For instance, a gap exists between the cortical and subcortical levels in the brain and between the deep and surface bodies. Indeed, Adrian Johnston[29] situates an initial gap within the brain itself. There are the unrepresented subcortical and affective structures and the neo-cortical declarative structures. According to him, the well-known Lacanian dictum *Il n'y pas de rapport sexuel*[30] (there is no sexual relationship) can then be supplemented by *Il n'y a pas de rapport intracérébral.* Complete alignment between the two levels is impossible. Ariane Bazan additionally points to a gap in our bodies, whereby vertebrates have *two* bodies. First is the deep body: a bag or tubular system of internal organs with smooth, involuntary muscles responsible for vegetative systems such as respiration, digestion, excretion and so on. More than five hundred million years ago, it was complemented by a surface body consisting of a skeleton and transverse muscles controlled precisely and voluntarily by specific brain structures.

Historicity

The deep and surface body coordination needs to be established mainly through experience. This applies to all vertebrates but is a fortiori to the human child, characterised as it is by extensive helplessness and dependence.[31] Hours after birth, the calf is teetering on its feet and knows how to find its mother's udder, but in our Western world, it can easily take more than twenty years before we can stand on our own two feet in the complete sense of the word.

In her essentially affirmative commentary on Solms' *The Conscious Id,* Bazan[32] introduces precision. Besides the brain, she says, we cannot do without the body as a place of origin. She quotes Freud: 'We have decided to associate pleasure and unpleasure with the quantity of excitation present – and in no way bound – in the soul's life, in such a way that unpleasure corresponds to an increase and pleasure to a decrease of this quantity'.[33] To Bazan, the decrease in tension that Freud calls pleasure comes from the body, not the brain. Only when an action or motor programme is successful will it lead to pleasure, resulting in reduced *bodily* tension. The behaviour producing relaxation is then physiologically marked as salient in our central nervous system. It is henceforth *worth repeating*.

What Kent Berridge[34] makes transparent can also be found in Freud.[35] Satisfaction must have been experienced before to trigger the need to repeat it. We should expect, according to Freud,[36] that nature would provide sufficiently secure predictions so that gratification would not be left to chance. Once a physiological marking occurs, exhibiting specific behaviour produces a dopamine surge because of the mesolimbic circuit (the pleasure nucleus or *nucleus accumbens*).[37] This pleasure indicates a particular *direction*. Thus, for an animal in captivity, only positing an *unnatural* behaviour (e.g. pressing a lever) will produce food. Then this act (however unnatural) will act as an *incentive*.

In this way, the dopaminergic mesolimbic system is a historicising system. It is not a priori clear which bodily action meets the alleviation of an internal need. Structurally, there is a lack of alignment between distress and behaviour. Even in animals, a movement pre-wired by instinct must be marked by dopamine release to be stored as *worth repeating*. The body continuously records a personal history of *contingent* events.[38] It responds to a system by which an action, independent of its outcome and independent of its object, can become pleasurable.

In this context, Bazan refers to the so-called *auto-shaping*.[39] If a grain appears in the feeder when a light is on, the pigeon – once conditioned – will start pecking at the feeder when the light goes on. If you introduce inconsistency and, in the second instance, sometimes offer a grain in the bowl and sometimes when the light is on and sometimes not, then something remarkable happens to the pigeon's behaviour. It starts pecking (not at the feeder but) at the *light*. This behaviour provides no nutritional benefit but indicates that the pecking motion's discharge is a relief. The pigeon allows itself to be fooled (although we might also say it becomes neurotic)! It is a fine example of how the link between the needs of the deep body and the behaviour of the surface body must be physiologically inscribed by an initial signal from the deep body indicating the tension was effectively reduced. Afterwards, however, the behaviour can (also) take on a life of its own. If the conduct were instrumental, the pigeon would stop pecking, but it cannot block its conditioned behaviour even after thousands of times. It is a phenomenon called self-maintenance (*auto-maintenance*)[40] that might be relevant to explaining the neuro-logic of repetition compulsion.

Drive and Affect

To French psychoanalyst Andre Green the affect is the signifier of the flesh and the flesh of the signifier.[41] From the perspective and according to the logic described, however, Bazan considers the drive a more primitive category than affect. Indeed, the drive first installs a mechanism of action determined by a history of events. This inscription is independent of the affective valence that it acquires only secondarily. Much more than animals, humans need the pleasure criterion of the deep body to lead to afferent excitation of the brainstem. Motor expression is, therefore, much less an a priori given than specific formulations by Solms (such as instincts as intrinsic emotional stereotypes) would suggest.[42]

The dopaminergic *incentive sensitisation*[43] compensates for the emergence of the surface body in vertebrates and becomes the driver of motor interaction with the outside world. The deep body and surface body have their logic, and a need arises for biological historiography to link needs to appropriate motor behaviour. This applies pre-eminently to the physiologically immature human child, who is not equipped to bind or discharge inner tension build-up. For this, the child ideally needs prolonged interaction with a big Other (usually the mother). Translated to Solms and Friston, each of us has to take stock *along the way* of which *prediction errors* are our own. It is a process mediated by *primary caretakers* or, in ordinary human language: the parents. Our first encounters (including with our bodies) are incomprehensible and inexplicable. At the outset, therefore, *prediction errors* are trumps. Building a predictive model for our bodies presupposes (in the total sense of the word) a necessary intervention of the big Other.

At the neuropsychoanalytic congress held in Mexico City in 2018, Ariane Bazan and colleagues presented some differences between drive and affect and did so based on similar findings in psychoanalysis, neuroscience and cognitive psychology.[44] Freud's initial theory revolves around pleasure. Discharge and tension relief are triggered there by an adequate act that, after all, leads to the satisfaction of a shortage at the origin of the drive.[45] Simply put: the child is hungry, cries, a big Other interprets, provides nourishment, there is tension release, this includes pleasure and crying as an – so it turns out – adequate (motor) activity leads to gratification and by itself allows for enjoyment/*jouissance*. According to Lacan,[46] this *jouissance* does not imply satisfaction of a need but of the drive. In a clinical context, he defines *jouissance* as the paradoxical satisfaction the subject experiences through his symptom. It is Freud's primary pathological gain; libido and *jouissance* are of the same order.[47] The gratification experience produces pleasure (thanks to consumption) and *jouissance* (the reward associated with bodily excitement). When a similar need arises, or we think we are approaching the Thing, the memory trace of a gratification experience is reactivated. This produces *jouissance* that is purely the result of motor tension. The memory of a mark that once created a *jouissance* revives this jouissance and installs a compulsion to repeat.

This division used by Bazan et al. between pleasure and *jouissance* parallels the neuroscientific distinction already made by Kent Berridge between LIKING and WANTING. LIKING revolves around subcortical opioid circuits.[48] It is expressed through facial expressions or behaviour manifesting themselves in different ways.[49] In contrast, WANTING is located in the mesolimbic dopamine circuits that ascend to the pleasure nucleus and prefrontal cortex. They involve the degree of motor activation the organism is willing to invest in obtaining a reward.

LIKING and pleasure provide the hedonic valence that people attribute to objects, ranging from positive or delicious to negative or aversive. *Jouissance* and WANTING are (only) expressed according to the intensity with which people respond[50] or the degree of their bodily activation.[51] Based on this finding, Bazan and Detandt[52] conclude that pleasure and *jouissance*, LIKING and WANTING differ from each other and that psychopathology results from the fact that specific motor patterns produce *jouissance* but (1) do not lead to pleasure, (2) are neither adequate nor satisfying and (3) on the other hand, may even be painful or harmful. *Jouissance* without pleasure and WANTING without LIKING align with what Berridge[53] argues is at play in addiction. Indeed, addictive behaviour persists despite harmful consequences and the absence of pleasure or even the presence of unpleasantness. The dopaminergic system does provide 'incentive salience' by increasing motivational or intentional value independently of any opioid-modulated 'good feeling' that once followed it.

In sum, throughout this view, *pleasure* is associated with consuming an object that satisfies a need. The thing is attractive or delicious. Pleasure results from tension reduction and restoration of homeostasis. We can share such experiences with others and communicate about them linguistically and by the facial expressions accompanying them. *Jouissance* is of a very different order. It is associated with a motor act that was (once) rewarded because it was adequate. This enjoyment results from tension increase that causes activation by the imposition of a need or the encounter with a stimulus that refers to the Thing. It belongs to the drive category, and it involves a combination of activity and alertness. It is 'mute'/dumb,[54] hidden or transgressive and cannot be inferred from facial expressions.

Pleasure and Enjoyment

Pleasure and enjoyment are distinct.[55] In Freud's theory of drives, pleasure is due to tension reduction that is, in turn, due to the consumption of an appropriate drive object. In contrast, Lacanian enjoyment (*jouissance*)[56] results from mobilising or utilising the body that was (once) adequate to satisfy the drive. Note that this description fits the legal origin of the term *jouissance*, namely that of usufruct. Pleasure is linked to the object, while enjoyment/jouissance is (merely) related to the motor act that leads (or has led) to it. According to this view, enjoyment and pleasure are different aspects of drive gratification. They correspond to the dopaminergic WANTING (Panksepp) and the opioid *LIKING* (Berridge) systems. They are respectively about libidinal pleasure as a wave of the drive (phenomenological: of wanting *something* – cf Panksepp's *a goad without a goal*) on which you ride and pleasure when this wave reaches its endpoint and comes to rest. As Lacan put it: '*Le plaisir fait barrière à la jouissance*'[57]: pleasure limits enjoyment.[58]

Enjoyment and pleasure are inextricably bound. Freud's pleasure, however, lies in the reduction of unpleasant tension. In this sense, the counterpart of the build-up of pressure (Freud's *Vor-Lust*) is precisely typical of enjoyment. They both belong to the drive category and correspond to the efficacy of a previous action. All this while affect (including hedonic affect: pleasant or unpleasant) is a secondary category assigned to the drive only *afterwards*. Bazan[59] gives the following example. In feeding and defecation, the motor movement, sucking and pressing, respectively, will quickly be re-tensioned later, producing enjoyment/pleasure. This enjoyment includes the promise of an expected pleasurable discharge. It accompanies any repeated tension increase that commemorates an inaugural event. It has its physiological counterpart in activating motor schedules by the dopaminergic mesolimbic circuitry.

We can presume a conglomeration of such seminal mechanisms in more complex psychosocial acts. They, too, acquire the same pleasure/dopaminergic incentive. Repetition similarly installs itself in the various symbolic-imaginary actions and interactions in clinical practice. What are they other than what Freud called fixations? The patient becomes absorbed in all sorts of actions or relationships that, on the face of it, bring him no benefit. Often quite the contrary.

Bazan[60] defines enjoyment pragmatically as what causes certain behaviours to be repeated even though they are not (or are no longer) beneficial or sometimes even harmful. Hence, to Lacan,[61] enjoyment is about 'satisfaction of the drive' and not that of the need (cf. Solms' *needs*). Enjoyment does have an evolutionary benefit or importance, namely that it helps to attune (the needs of) the inner body to (the actions of) the outer body.

And what if we look at drive and affect or pleasure and enjoyment in the context of our sexual life? Some drives are vital and linked to the needs of the deep body, but sexual urges are very different, as one can safely survive without sex. Freud[62] states that besides a 'drive', a nature in itself non-sexual, arising from sources of motor impulses, one distinguishes ... a contribution from a stimulus-receiving organ (skin, mucous membrane, sense organ). The latter is to be considered here as an erogenous[63] zone, as the organ whose excitation gives the drive its sexual character'.

Freud[64] talks about the Ego- or self-preservative drives versus the sexual drive, and Lacan (as described earlier) distinguished between need, demand and desire. Somewhat simplified, these are, respectively, (1) the need for real and energetic-material satisfaction, (2) the demand for (the imaginary of) expressions of love and (3) finally, there is the (eminently human) desire. This desire belongs to the symbolic order. It is characterised (like a dream) by mechanisms such as condensation and displacement, and it is directed towards 'It' that is never 'That': something that (to you) is never the real Thing.[65] I am reminded of Lacan's famous statement: '*l'amour, c'est donner ce qu'on n'a pas*'.[66] The beloved keeps a treasure hidden inside. Some Things cannot be put into words and yet they are what the loved one 'has' or 'gives'. To this enigmatic object, small a, all romantic love owes its alchemy.[67] If it's right, it begins as bliss, and it doesn't become (too) messy in the end.[68]

The next question is: what do affect, drive, pleasure, and enjoyment have to do with sex? Freud[69] would possibly call the dynamics we have described either pre-genital, the drives for self-preservation or drives in a general sense. They are ultimately linked to the basic needs of the deep body, and, as explained, they may involve pleasure and enjoyment, but that in itself is not enough to call them sexual. Following the previous Freud quote, Bazan[70] suggests the category of the sexual specifically comes about as the pleasurable at the level of the so-called 'erogenous zones'. She initially proposes a mechanical or logical definition of what qualifies for erogenous zone status. In particular, these are the edges or openings of the body where the deep and surface body is in direct contact, such as the oral cavity, anus, genitals or nipples.

To Bazan, *The Essence of Sex*[71] sprouts historically from the direct stimulation of erogenous zones and is also bound up with the enjoyment of this act. Thus, it leads to the creation of accidental/contingent objects inherent to the narrative of the particular subject. A specific *subject* that, through a dynamic inherent in a linguistic operation, can become an *object*.[72] Elsewhere, then, I have elaborated in detail how and why human sexuality (in a neologism borrowed from Joyce McDougall)[73] is always *neo-sexuality*. In the statistics of the Gauss curve, very many positions are possible.[74] All sexuality is a collage or *bricolage*[75] of partial drives and (traumatic or pleasurable) events.

The non-sexual remains entirely dependent on the need satisfaction of the depth-body. It does not lead to the constitution of truly representational objects. The objects of need are (real/energetic-material) substances whose action remains beyond the reach of representation for the subject undergoing them. Referring to Bazan,[76] linguistic reversals are impossible for the 'objects' of need because of their physiological and necessary anchoring. This, while creating pleasure in thinking of oneself as an object (as it comes up in many sexual fantasies or scenarios), can only be the structural outcome of a specific sexual dynamic.

Following each event, motor patterns are dopaminergically inscribed in the body's history. For the erogenous zones, it is then the action itself – that is, the direct touching of these zones – that brings about the event: in particular, it is the action of the surface body that directly touches the deep body. In contrast to the parameters (such as air or food) of the deep body, there is a physiological homeostasis absent in the sex. In this sense, no 'adequate act' is possible at the level of the erogenous zones. You cannot survive without air, but you can survive without sex. Solms' needs have a homeostatic criterion, and in terms of pre-genital drive-objects, there is a certain generalisability. At the same time, both the purpose and object of the sexual drive remain radically contingent and can be sublimated.

Repetition

Even when it concerns the demonic of the unconscious, it affects not in the least *repetition*.[77] The patient knows what he should think and how to feel or act. Everyone (including many 'professionals') tries to make him understand or teach him the *right* thoughts, feelings and behaviours. Still, he comes up against a repetition of unwanted thoughts, feelings or behaviour (in endless variations on the same theme). In other words, the reality of the clinic constantly contradicts adaptation, the pleasure principle and (the pursuit of) constancy or homeostasis. These may be consciously pursued, but the rationale does not match persistent 'irrational' forces. In this context, I like to quote Aristotle, to whom this statement is attributed: we are what we repeatedly do. And wasn't it Einstein who defined folly as follows: always doing the same thing and expecting a different result?

You can repeat without knowing or realising *that* you are repeating. This is the repetition Freud talks about in one of his clinical writings: *Remembering, Repeating and Working Through*.[78] Both enactment and transference can be considered forms of such repetition.[79] First, you have to find out *whether* you repeat, then *what* you repeat, and finally, you have to try to remember where and when this pattern of repetition took root. Not that this would solve the matter in itself. Another long and arduous phase of working through comes next. But there's also a kind of repetition, where you know and realise that and even *what* you are repeating. This may be the case in post-traumatic repetition.

In lesson 28 of his *Introductory Lectures* of 1917, Freud described how traumatic neurosis results from fixation on a traumatic event. Patients repeat the traumatic situation in their dreams. In the process, they are catapulted back to the past. It is as if the patient has not finished with the trauma. There is, as it were, an urgent task left to him that has not yet been completed. Thus, soldiers' post-traumatic dreams do not respond at all to the pleasure principle, which, after all, aims to reduce tension. However, according to Freud, unconsciously repeating traumatic events or symptoms would help them master pain and emotional conflict. The post-traumatic dream serves another task that must be completed before the pleasure principle can establish its dominance. Such dreams try to retroactively master the stimulus and still develop a (protective signalling) fear that was lacking during trauma.

In *Beyond the Pleasure Principle* from 1920, this train of thought is further elaborated based on the stimulus shield (*Reizschutz*) breached in response to a traumatic experience because the excitations are too great to be captured and psychically bound. The psychic apparatus regresses to more primitive modes of reaction. The perception of time is disturbed because it collapses. Severe trauma unleashes the death drive or dissolving forces. Turning passive into active, on the other hand, provides a kind of 'pleasure'. In the repetition compulsion, the trauma comes into a *replay*. It is an attempt to bind the trauma psychologically so that it can be engaged in the narrative (Lacanian: the chain of signifiers), and the reign of the pleasure principle can re-establish itself.

In *Inhibitions, Symptoms and Anxiety* from 1926, Freud describes the Ego in trauma as being utterly helpless in the face of excruciating excitation. While the Ego would generally produce an anxiety signal on time when danger is imminent, in trauma, it is overwhelmed by automatic, that is, traumatic anxiety. Incidentally, such traumatic anxiety can arise due to an excessive drive or external events. Freud could never define precisely the relationship between external events and internal processes. What does concern him decisively, however, is the *too much*: an outsized stimulus and a paralysed Ego that no longer manages to discharge the accumulated tension nor to bind it to psychic representations. Paul Verhaeghe[80] would later talk about *structural* trauma caused by the drive-impulse versus *accidental* trauma resulting from an event occurring in reality.

Ariane Bazan points out that many studies have shown that *every* surprise leads to a dopamine spike in the pleasure nucleus or *nucleus accumbens*. Not only pleasant experiences are marked by it, but also a variety of unpleasant, disgusting, stressful or painful events. It is not the hedonistic valence that matters but the event content *by itself* that exerts its effect. The organism is surprised; the body is unexpectedly stirred. The dopamine spike then causes the actions the organism had actively displayed in the vicinity of this unanticipated event to be ratified. This *incentive salience* causes action patterns to be naturally inscribed. Molecular and cellular changes occur. As a result, they are triggered faster, easier and more forcefully each time. Behold the neuronal that she believes underlies repetition.

Repetition Compulsion

Freud introduced the concept of repetition compulsion at sixty-four, thus relatively late in his clinical and theoretical development. In his words, it lies beyond the pleasure principle[81] but may *precede* this principle. Moreover, Bazan devotes much more attention to this phenomenon than Mark Solms. It seems to breach the fundamental assumption of homeostasis and the pursuit of minimal tension.[82] In his *Logique du Fantasme,* Lacan[83] argues that this repetition only establishes a truly *subjective* regime categorically different from the homeostatic pleasure principle.

Bazan further aligns herself with Lacan when she names the repetition compulsion a conceptual intrusion (*'intrusion conceptuelle'*) of great magnitude. A few years later, she states:[84] 'What Freud deals with in 1920 when exploring the unconscious is repetition. Repetition (…) is the precise designation of a mark (German: *Zug*) (…) insofar as it recalls the eruption of enjoyment' To Lacan, this repetition is constitutive of the mind as a specific matter. According to him, we cannot do without it if we are to do justice (Lacan: *'faire valoir'*)[85] to what Freud was really after: the subject of the unconscious or the unconscious subject with its very characteristic module of the compulsion to repeat.

About this repetition, psychoanalysis classically refers to the *fort/da* game played and replayed by Freud's grandson Ernst Wolfgang at the age of eighteen months. Freud described and interpreted it in the second chapter of his *Beyond the Pleasure Principle*. In that period (immediately after the First World War), he was fully occupied with the traumatic, that is war neurosis (today called post-traumatic stress disorder or PTSD). How can we understand that in these kinds of problems, the patient repeatedly goes into the same painful states of mind and behaviours? Karl Abraham even spoke of traumatophilia in this context[86]: the (at first sight altogether) incomprehensible phenomenon of the traumatised person showing a kind of predilection for traumatising experiences.

Freud's grandson Ernst Wolfgang was a quiet and well-behaved little boy with no complaints or symptoms who hardly cried when his mother left him alone for several hours. What was remarkable was that he would take visible pleasure in throwing all kinds of small objects into the corner of the room or under the bed. This act was accompanied by an 'oh oh oh', a sound both his mother and Grandpa Freud interpreted as *fort* ('away') and which Ernst also uttered whenever he played peekaboo with his mirror image. Little Ernst experienced great satisfaction from his power over the disappearance of the object (or of himself). Later Freud observed his grandson flinging a bobbin beyond his field of vision only to *tirelessly* pull it back into view by its string, accompanied by a joyous exclamation *da* (there!).

Should the Ernst of play be understood as a way of mastering painful experiences (in this case of separation)? Does turning passive into active (as it often does in many children's games) play a leading role? If the doctor has carried out a nasty throat exam or a painful procedure, we can almost be sure these elements will recur in the affected child's play later. It exchanges the passive position of reality for the active part of play/fantasy, simultaneously passing on the unpleasant experience to his playmate and avenging him on someone innocent. From everyday life: a little boy gets beaten up at school and begins to harass his pet at home (although he loves it very much… with all the guilt this entails).

However, the main problem for Freud is the contradiction in this scene between the repetition of compulsion and the pleasure principle.[87] What satisfaction could result from repeating actions that had initially caused unpleasant feelings? Freud explains that in his play, the child discovers a way of mastering by *binding* tensions through motor action: flinging away and pulling back while repeating (and thus motor articulating) oh and ah, *fort* and *da*. This simultaneously creates a release of tension and relinquishment of raw drive gratification. Using the (still proto-mental) primal signifiers oh and ah detaches the drive from the (un-)pleasurable aspects of the experience.

Lacan links the *fort-da* game to the operation of the symbolic order. In his view, Ernst neutralises above all the real or traumatic impact by constructing a *representation* of it. This representation is symbolically articulated because it is based on the difference between two signifiers picked up from the big Other: *fort* and *da*. Thus, he imposes a pattern of predictability on a separation he is otherwise at the mercy of. Every time Ernst makes the bobbin disappear, he relishes the anticipation of being able to make it re-appear. The word *fort* is a *présence faite d'absence*[88]: a presence made of an absence. The disappeared/absent bobbin persists in psychic reality thanks to a signifier that guarantees its symbolic survival. This ultimately binary off/on or 0/1 provides an order according to which predictability or laws arise. As such, the *fort-da* game is constitutive of true mental life. It is governed as much by repetition as by homeostasis or the pleasure principle.

Once a well-defined action has been linked to an event, the motivation for this action becomes separated from the gratification of the drive itself. The relaxation of tension resulting from the satisfaction of a need originating in the deep body is purely incidental to or contingent on the action the surface body has undertaken. Tension and relaxation are a by-product. They are essential for survival but not determinative of repetitive behaviour. Regardless of the outcome, the child will endlessly repeat: both (for example) his sucking and his tireless *fort* and *da*. Bazan[89] formulates this in a single sentence: '*It is from within the repetition compulsion that relief of tension becomes possible – it is not the relief of tension that is the ground for repetition*'.

Endnotes

1   Bazan (2017) researched the Lacanian signifier using the tachistoscope. This is an instrument that shows an image for an ultra-short time. It can be used as a training tool to increase recognition speed, show something so briefly that it is not consciously registered, or investigate which elements are remembered/retained by memory. To Lacan, the unconscious is dynamic and linguistically structured around signifiers. The signifier is primarily a phonological object with different meanings depending on the context. It can carry an emotional charge that triggers mental activity outside the knowing/consciousness of the person involved. Alpha synchronisation is the synchronous pattern of slow

brain waves (8–12 Hz) that is defensive against stimuli causing internal conflict. See also Shevrin (2010) and Shevrin et al. (2013) as well as Shevrin et al. (1996).

2 Salas et al. (2021).
3 Nietzsche (1980 [1878]).
4 How does a subject respond after a prior (in this case, subliminal, i.e. descriptively unconscious) stimulus?
5 Bazan (2017).
6 De Saussure (2002 [1916]).
7 Ibid., p. 66.
8 Lacan (1981b, p. 263).
9 Lacan (–2006 [1957]).
10 Bazan (2007a, 2011b), Kinet (2008a).
11 Freud (1909a, 1909b). The Rat Man was a man with obsessive-compulsive symptoms. He feared rats would bore into his anus (he had heard of such torture practices). The signifier 'rat' played a prominent role in his story. Other famous examples of the signifier game include Freud's analysis of the *Käfer/Que faire*. Where a phonetic, that is, signifier logic, also operates. In his letter to Fliess of 29/12/1897, he calls this logic (Yiddish) *Meshugge* i.e. crazy. Still, Freud's genius lies not least in the fact that he could distil the secrets of the human mind precisely from its waste products (dream, parapraxis).
12 Bazan (2002, 2006, 2007b). Very recently, Olyff and Bazan (2023) conducted another pervasive and impressive experiment in which, after priming, the signifier's phonology (and not the semantics) turned out to be decisive. Their conclusions are that the ambiguous phonological translation of the world influences our mental processing without us being aware of this influence … The results show that the images induced inadvertent rebus priming in naive participants. In other words, our results show that people solve rebuses unwittingly independent of stimulus order, constituting empirical evidence for the mental effects of the signifier.
13 Lacan (1986, p. 158). Derrida (1988, p. 252).
14 Bazan (2005, 2010, 2011b).
15 Peirce (1994).
16 I elaborate on the apple, which was used as an example by Bazan (2014b). To have or to be the phallus is (after all) nothing other than to have or to be the apple of the (m-) other's eye.
17 Sartre (1996 [1946]) see earlier note. One of the main existentialist premises is that in man *l'existence précède l'essence.* Existence precedes essence.
18 See also Slavoj Žižek (1989, pp. 184–185), where he calls the object small a the pure void which functions as the object-cause of desire.
19 Bowen-Moore (1989).
20 In Dutch, '*appel*' means apple, but it is also a demand for help (an appeal) addressed to the other.
21 The distinction between science and poetry is central in Robert Collingwood's (1933) *An essay on philosophical method.* In science, definitions of terms are essential. Its concepts need transparent and hard edges. This is in dramatic contrast to poetry, where words are stretched and expanded so that we are forced to look at them afresh. Ambiguity makes poetry flourish. See the next chapter.
22 Lacan (1953a, p. 259).
23 Fink (1997).
24 Kinet (2002). '*Le symbole est le meurtre de la Chose*' (Lacan 1966, p. 319). The symbol murders the Thing (my translation) For discussion of the Thing, see also Kinet (2002, 2017)
25 Freud (1912).
26 Harmful or deadly not only because of non-adaptive but also because of *punishment* for breaking the *law*.

27 Lacan sometimes calls them *béance*, sometimes *déhiscence fondamentale* or *discord primordial*. For those who want to delve into this complicated matter, I would like to refer to Verhaeghe (2001). Paraphrasing Nietzsche, by leaping from (the imaginary identification with) the mirror stage, we become masters of our own chaos. See next note.

28 Nobus (1998), Lacan (1949). The *infans* has poor motor coordination due to the delay in developing its central nervous system. In this sense, every child is born prematurely. Lacan speaks of the law of the heart (*la loi du coeur*, 1950, p. 174): the desire to create an order out of chaos and the desire to conceive a self as a controllable unit. He calls it an insane (*insensée*) undertaking because the subject misses in chaos the true manifestation of his being (*être actuel*, ibid., pp. 171–172). There is a gap between *le Moi (m'aître/m'être)* and *être*. This gap is closed by the symbolic-imaginary. Intimate connections between body and world emerge that last throughout our lives. On the one hand, a child sees in the outside world nothing but images of its corporeality; on the other, it learns to represent and animate the outside world through its body. All of (post-) Kleinian thought, to Lacanians, revolves around the imaginary colonisation of that first outside world: the maternal body. Lacan reads their transference-countertransference continuum as a dual (imaginary) relation, which he believes the analyst must renounce. To Lacan, the analyst primarily has a symbolic function. He juxtaposes against the countertransference the desire of the analyst. This desire continues to acknowledge the lack and thus avoids what he considers to be the imaginary trap of adaptation.

29 Johnston (2013).

30 Several Lacanian 'slogans' are constantly circulating worldwide. *L'Autre de l'Autre n'existe pas*. The Other of the Other doesn't exist. *LA femme n'existe pas*. THE woman *doesn't exist*. *Il n'y a pas de rapport sexuel*. *There is no sexual relationship* and so on. The latter, of course, does not mean that no sexual relationship(s) exist but that due to the linguistic nature of human psychosexuality, no Jack has a 'natural' Jill. In everyday life: we fall in love with someone we *don't* know, and we divorce someone we *do* know.

31 Bazan (2007b, 2016).

32 Bazan (2013, p. 20).

33 Freud (1920a, 1920b).

34 Berridge (2009), Berridge, Robinson and Aldridge (2010).

35 Freud (1905a, p. 66, 1905b, p. 182).

36 Ibid.

37 Schultz (1998).

38 In his seminar on the four fundamental concepts of psychoanalysis, Lacan (1973) discusses the contingency (*tuchè*) of the real and the regularities (*automaton*) of the symbolic-imaginary whose other-worldly causality plays a role in all psycho-(patho-)-logy. See also Aguiar (2018).

39 Di Ciano et al. (2001) in Bazan (2016a).

40 Killeen (2003).

41 Bazan (2017, note 21).

42 Robinson and Berridge (1993, 2000, 2003), Berridge (2007).

43 Fotopoulou and Tsakiris (2017).

44 Freud (1915e, f).

45 Lacan (1986).

46 Lacan (1991b).

47 Berridge (2009).

48 Robinson and Berridge (1993).

49 Berridge (1996).

50 Bradley and Lang (1994).

51 Verschuere, Crombez and Koster (2001).

52 Bazan and Detandt (2013).

53 Berridge (2009).
54 In Dutch *'stom'* means mute *and* dumb/stupid. Cf an earlier note quoting Freud on the silence/muteness of the death drive.
55 Bazan and Detandt (2013).
56 Some more words on *jouissance*. It is an original and key concept from Lacanian psychoanalysis and literally means (in a notary context) usufruct. It is usually left untranslated, although some call it enjoyment. Only after 1960 did it evolve into a concept of its own, distinct from pleasure. The pleasure principle limits enjoyment, it limits *jouissance* and paradoxically commands the subject to enjoy as little as possible. *Jouissance*, conversely, involves a constant tendency to exceed this law or limit and go beyond the pleasure principle. The result then is not a surplus of pleasure but rather pain. The prohibition of *jouissance* is inherent in the symbolic structure of language. Moreover, our entry into the symbolic order depends on a certain initial renunciation of *jouissance* in the context of the castration complex. In it, the subject gives up his attempt to be the imaginary phallus of the mother. He thus withdraws from and protects himself from the enjoyment of the (first) big Other who uses him (incestuously) as fruit. *Jouissance*, according to Lacan, paves the path to death (Lacan 1991b, p. 17). Its impossible enjoyment seems (only) forbidden. Insofar as the drive is an attempt in search of *jouissance* by breaking the pleasure principle every drive is a death drive. Towards the end of his teaching, Lacan (1975b) further distinguishes between phallic *jouissance* and feminine *jouissance*, which he also calls the enjoyment of the big Other. The former bears resemblance to Freud's (regarded as masculine) libido, the latter is supplementary, is unbounded and lies beyond the phallus (ibid., p. 69) in unmentionable and unspeakable ways. I will end this note with a Lacanian formula: *Jouissance* + *Nom du Père* = *Principe de Plaisir*. I try to obey Shakespeare: brevity is the soul of wit.
57 Lacan (1994, p. 22).
58 In *Subversion of the subject and the dialectic of desire in the Freudian Unconscious* Lacan (1960) affirms that it is not the law that bars the subject's access to *jouissance*. It is pleasure.
59 Bazan (2015, 2016a).
60 Bazan (2015, 2016a), Bazan and Detandt (2013, 2015).
61 Lacan (1986, pp. 244–248).
62 Freud (1905a, p. 97, 1905b, p. 224).
63 In the pre-genital phase, pleasure is experienced by stimulating erogenous zones such as skin, mouth and anus. Much of this is included in foreplay or falls prey to repression (Freud 1905a, p. 85). Only in the genital phase does the emphasis shift to the pubic or bikini region.
64 Freud (1905a, 1905b, 1915e, 1915f).
65 Kinet (2002, 2018).
66 In full: *à quelqu'un qui n'en veut pas*, i.e. to someone who doesn't want it (nor wants to know anything about it) (Lacan 1994, p. 151).
67 In his VIII Seminar on transference Lacan (1991a) elaborates extensively on Plato's *Symposium* and its different viewpoints on love. Alcibiades is in love with the ugly Socrates. He desires Socrates because he presumes Socrates is in possession of the *agalma* (a hidden treasure). There is no rapport between what the loved one/ Socrates *'possesses'* and what the loving one/Alcibiades *'lacks'*. This inescapable deadlock defines the loved one: the other sees some Thing in me and wants some Thing from me, but I cannot give what I do not possess. A genuine love can only emerge when I am not simply/only fascinated by the *agalma* in the other, but when I experience the other as frail and lost, as lacking *'it'* and when my love manages to survive this loss.

68 In common parlance, it is all about the honeymoon. Lyrically and according to Victor Hugo: *Qu'est-ce que des amants? Ce sont des nouveau-nés.* My translation: What are lovers? They are new-borns. In a more graphic guise (and according to a famous Hollywood movie), bliss lasts *9 1/2 Weeks.*

69 Freud (1905a, 1915e, 1915f).

70 Bazan (2015).

71 Ibid.

72 See, for example, all the ubiquitous passive-active reversals in BDSM.

73 Kinet (2011b).

74 Kinet (2015a, 2015b).

75 Strauss (1962)

76 Bazan (2015, 2016a), which I largely paraphrase here.

77 Lacan (1973) argues in his XI Seminar that repetition is one of the four fundamental concepts of psychoanalysis

78 Freud (1914a, 1914b).

79 Repetition stems from two forces: automatism on the side of the signifier and the missed encounter with the object/Thing on the part of the drive. Lacan uses the term 'insistence' to name the repetition characteristic of the signifying chain in the unconscious. The Lacanian unconscious is neither primordial nor instinctual. In his text *The Agency of the Letter in the Unconscious* (1957), he defines the unconscious as a memory system like that of the (then) modern thinking machines where the signifying chain insists on reproducing. In his Seminar on *La relation d'objet* 1956-1957 (1994) he elaborates on the paradoxical function of transference within the psychoanalytic treatment. In its symbolic aspect, repetition helps the cure progress by revealing the signifiers of the subject's history. The imaginary (love and hate) aspect acts as resistance.

80 Verhaeghe (2017).

81 Freud (1920a, 1920b).

82 Lacan (1966a).

83 Lacan (2017b, p. 134).

84 Lacan (1991a, pp. 88–89).

85 Lacan (2017, p. 280).

86 Abraham (1907).

87 He postulates the death drive (Thanatos) in addition to the life drive (Eros). One must say that the concept is and remains very controversial within psychoanalysis. For an excellent critical review, I refer to Jens De Vleminck (2014). The death drive introduced by Freud in 1920 is mainly imitated in the (post-) Kleinian and Lacanian developments, but each case receives its interpretation. While the former mainly include aggressive, destructive or envious tendencies, with Lacan, the death drive becomes the fundamental tendency to produce repetition because of the symbolic order. In other words, the death drive loses its natural roots with him. It must be distinguished from the biological tendency to return to the dead matter of the inorganic state. Towards the end of his teaching, Lacan even considers the death drive as an aspect of every drive. Every drive is a virtual death drive because every drive is destructive, repetitive and excessive. It seeks its extinction, drive relates to a repetitive subject, and drive is an attempt (beyond the pleasure principle) to enter the realm of excessive *jouissance* where enjoyment becomes painful (and sometimes even deadly). A recognisable example is the intoxication-bringing ecstasy of passion or addiction.

88 '*Le mot est déjà une présence faite d'absence*'. The word is a presence made of absence. (Lacan 1966, p. 276).

89 Bazan and Detandt (2017, p. 7).

Chapter 18

Interlude

A Clinical Objective Correlative?

I will start with the enigmatic opening verses from one of the twentieth century's most famous English-language poems, *The Waste Land,* by poet and Nobel Prize for Literature laureate T. S. Eliot.[1] Through what at first glance appears just a description of seasons and situations, the reader is led imperceptibly into a very personal mental universe. It is generally agreed that the decay of civilisation and the hopelessness of existence are galvanised in it.

More theoretically, Eliot introduced the concept of the objective correlative in literary criticism.[2] This implies that, according to him, there is only one right way to express an emotion in a work of art. The artist must use a set of subjects, situations or events as the formula for a private feeling. He does this in such a way that these external elements lead to a sensation that immediately evokes the emotion in question. Eliot's imagistic poetry can be read as a sequence of objective correlatives.

The term objective correlative came to mind during my intake interview with Helena. She was in her forties, simultaneously bright and frail, and consulted me due to complaints of anxiety and depression. Shortly before her birth, her grandmother on her father's side had hanged herself. She had always known this had been a burden to her father. It was as if the desperate spirit of his depressed mother had continued to haunt his mind. He could often be very absent-minded, and she often found him crying silently and alone in his studio. Helena's mother went from hard of hearing to deaf at a young age. An older brother was a scoundrel who never cared about anything or anyone. She was sturdy and a perfectionist. She tried to be both an angel and a ray of sunshine in the house. In a sense, she had always been a nurse and eventually became one professionally.

As is often the case with parentification,[3] she was too weighed down by caregiving duties for several years and ended 'below zero'. She calls herself highly sensitive. As an example, she recounts a memory. As a child, she would often lie awake. She could not sleep because she heard strange noises from the neighbour's basement. This worried her. How many times did she indicate this to her roommates? She could almost have yelled 'murder' or 'fire', but they would not have heard her. After all, her roommates didn't hear or notice anything. Only many years later, new tenants who had moved into the neighbouring house noticed the annoying clicking of the central heating boiler.

DOI: 10.4324/9781003394358-18

Some forms of parentification touch on secondary traumatisation. In the ordinary course of events, the parents act like an oyster whose mother-of-pearl produces layers around the grain of sand of the Lacanian real. Such a shell makes a difference. It is Bion's contact barrier as a kind of mental skin. Drive and trauma are remedied/mediated through this parental contribution. Their symbolic developmental assistance dampens, and waves of affect become more and better regulated.

Conversely, the child may have to mobilise its mental apparatus to metabolise drive and trauma originating from the parents. The child responds to the unconscious and unspoken needs of the parents and tries to parry or repair them. If necessary, it has or develops extra feelers or a sixth sense. It can maintain or safeguard the peace and security needed by timely intervention or anticipation. It is the identification with the aggressor as described not by Anna Freud but by Sandor Ferenczi[4] before her. The child responds proactively (and not reactively) to needs or expectations it assumes in an unsafe Other.

I gave Helena's memory a highly relevant status from our first conversation. As a child, she lay listening with pricked ears to the sounds from the neighbour's basement, which was an objective correlative. Her perception of the outer world reflected her inner world. It indicated how attuned she was to her parents' unconscious needs. She was preoccupied with the sounds in their basement. In her, all this had led to the formation of what Winnicott considers a False Self that was bound to fail sooner or later.

Helena went through a long period of clinical psychotherapy. For months, she was distraught, anxious, clamouring and appealing for intensive care. The amount of her suffering in the verbal therapies and contacts was, on the other hand, matched by her immense joy in creative expression in our art studio. The latter is at the heart of our ward. It is run by an artist (not therapeutically trained) who exerts a muse's influence and inspires everyone.

Now that Helena is in outpatient psychotherapy and back at work, she can indulge herself with clay. She dreams of making her own beautiful and warm (rather than cold and industrial) urns for the remains of cremated people and pets. She is looking everywhere for forms that fit these contents as 'moulded' as possible. Death, after all, requires an appropriate container. She has made a virtue of her 'high-sensitivity' need through sublimation and sinthome[5]: an urn for her grandmother, so she would no longer need to inhabit and crush her father. In her words: 'My view on things is not like that of the average person'. And then, smiling with half a wink: 'Thank goodness'.

Endnotes

1 Eliot (2002 [1922]). For *The Waste Land* on the Internet, see https://poets.org/poem/waste-land
2 Eliot (2004 [1951]).
3 Kinet (2010a).
4 Ferenczi (1982 [1933]).
5 The *sinthome* is a neologism coined by Lacan (2005). It is the creative invention of an idiosyncratic *jouissance*/enjoyment of a particular subject (Verhaeghe & Declercq 2002, p. 68).

Chapter 19

Finale

From the Poetic Child

Like the poet, Freud's grandson Ernst Wolfgang (and by extension every child) plays with signifiers as if they were objects.[1] They are essentially *mental* objects: words and images, sounds and symbols. To him, they even become *the* objects by which he discovers, expands and expresses his subjective universe. According to Walter Schönau,[2] poetry is an anthropological universal. It is of all times and all cultures. According to him, this observation provides a decisive argument for seeking the origins of poetry in our ontogenetic prehistory. Let me take some licence for a poetic excursion.[3]

From birth, the child is surrounded by his mother tongue. All his experiences are embedded in *basso continuo*, a murmur of language. Long before he understands the meaning of words, the child senses that words mean something, and he is confronted with their enigmatic *abracadabra*. From the beginning, this language also means a lot in an affective-existential sense, where it is not so much *what* but *that* and *how* things are said. The mother mirrors, modulates, and imitates. By tuning in to her child,[4] she provides affects with image, sound and rhythm. This enables evenemental encounters (cf. Daniel Stern's '*moments of meeting*')[5] that are emotionally highly meaningful. They form, as it were, so many stones to step on.

Without knowing it themselves, both mother and child honour a principle of Alexander Pope[6]: 'The sound must seem an echo to the sense'. According to poet and Nobel laureate T. S. Eliot, there is grasping without understanding, and communication without comprehension, characteristic of poetry.[7] That poetry is paradoxically associated with meaningfulness is, therefore, remarkable. After all, the poem is often not or only partially understood. Yet, it can trigger violent emotional reactions in us, comparable, for instance, to the effect of Portuguese fados, which move us to tears without us understanding an iota of the text.

This tendency towards meaninglessness has also been called the scandal of poetry.[8] Poetry does actual violence to language. It does not conform to the norm. It breaks the parlando of everyday speech by producing an enigmatic signifier or one signifier too many, here and there. On the one hand, it says something about the lack of a signifier, about not yet/no longer knowing what to say and saying

DOI: 10.4324/9781003394358-19

it. On the other hand, this chosen signifier captures the signified better than any other![9]Poetry arises anyway from a *manque-à-dire*. Paradoxically, it is a kind of non-verbal expression!

Baby language, *motherese* and poetic language all deviate from everyday language. The meaning cannot be fathomed. The language is not referential but associative. It is not discursive, not pragmatic. Just as the body is used purely expressively and not instrumentally in dance, so the poet dances with language. Language is an end in itself; its form is central. With a dowsing rod, the child and poet seek (in an encounter with the real of Thing, drive and trauma) the 'right' word, the word they want to find or invent. According to Jacques Lacan, an allusion to sublimation is about elevating a signifier to the dignity of the Thing.[10] This signifier is always (as the Dadaists called it) a ready-made or *objet trouvé*. It is fundamentally obtained from the big Other.

According to Flemish modernist Paul Van Ostaijen,[11] the poet throws words up and plays with them until they land on their feet. The poet is then a magician, a juggler and a lion tamer with a biro who tames desire and makes it jump through his flaming hoops. Words that might be chosen independently of their meaning and for the sake of their sonority function as transitional objects. Objects that represent the transition from a state of fusion with the mother to a different form: entering into a relationship with the mother as outside, as distinct. Words that, according to Donald Winnicott,[12] allow one to break free from the pre-logical and pre-verbal fusion of object and subject.

I refer to Van Ostaijen's most famous poem: *Mark greets things in the morning.*[13] In this poem, he introduces a little guy who first says 'hi' to some of his household items and eventually says 'goodbye' to a picture of a fisherman with a hat and a pipe. There are onomatopoeia and (part-)neologisms, with which the child/poet tries to grasp the Thing, but in vain. Signifiers take the upper hand and establish a new form of being sketched by Lacan's symbolic order, aka his big Other.

To the Neuropsychoanalytic Prose

To return to neuropsychoanalytic prose, these (again: *articulated*) motor actions are not to be adequate to be repeated. Indeed, they fundamentally fail in some sense. Bazan[14] laconically states that praying or singing does not help in case of an earthquake. Nor, for that matter, does the more mundane whistling in the dark. Yet, these actions are repeated. Ernst's *fort-da* has no impact on the coming and going of his mother but is nevertheless happily and triumphantly repeated. Bazan argues in purely Freudian terms that even if the act 'mis-grasps' the Thing rather than grasping it, this is still better than anxious dismay. After all, it is the repeated act *itself* that produces relief. This brings us to trauma.

In a very concise definition, we can economically characterise trauma as a sudden stimulus increase (Freud: *Erregung-Zuwachs*)[15] that overwhelms the mental apparatus, which cannot comprehend or 'contain' it. In the absence of a representation, the mental device cannot bind or channel it.[16] Traumatic or automatic anxiety is free energy that engulfs the subject just as the disintegration of the Ego exposes the subject to (the dissolution or dissipation of) entropy. Very characteristic of traumatic neurosis or post-traumatic stress disorder, on the other hand, are painful flashbacks, revivals and nightmares. They are concrete and raw (because they are undigested) regurgitations showing that all kinds of physical or sensory sensations have become etched, as they were, on the retina and other membranes.[17] In addition, there is constant, heightened vigilance. After all, both the inner and outer worlds are minefields. Flight or immobility seem to be the only resort. Tragically, it often happens that the victim repeatedly puts himself in traumatising situations. To make matters worse, he may even become a perpetrator or criminal (or feel he is) because involuntary passive-active reversals occur when a traumatic scene or relationship pattern is repeated with altered roles. In the latter case, we speak of enactment (German: *agieren*). The person involved does not remember anything but acts it out. He does not produce a memory but repetition without, of course, realising he is repeating.[18] Resistance then expresses itself through the repetition of actions.[19]

Now, many studies have shown that every surprise leads to a dopamine spike.[20] Not only are pleasant experiences marked by it but also a variety of unpleasant, disgusting, stressful or painful events. So it is not the hedonistic valence that matters, but the *event* content *in itself* that exerts its effect. The organism is surprised; the body is unexpectedly stirred. The dopamine spike then causes the actions (that the organism had actively displayed in the vicinity of this unanticipated event) to be ratified. This incentive salience[21] causes action patterns to be neurally inscribed. Molecular and cellular changes occur. As a result, they are triggered faster, more efficiently and forcefully every time.

Bazan suggests that any trauma-related action or behaviour is inherently better than mere passivity, numbness or freezing. Even if this action yields nothing in avoiding trauma, it is advantageous for the affected person to discharge body tension in a motor pattern because this (cf. see Karl Friston's *free energy principle*) at least reduces anxiety and free energy. Every motor action (including articulation) produces at least some form of discharge and represents structural gain compared to an excess of unbound tension. Lacan[22] also points to this fact: being *able* to dream is important for binding energy.[23] This is in line with what Wilfred Bion and other (post-)Kleinians say about the ability to dream, which has a healthy, protective function in its own right.

Finale

With this repetition and with the signifier, I will conclude my train of thought. According to Bazan, Freud already distinguished two things: to grasp/comprehend (in this case: a concept) and to mark it.[24] The first corresponds to the programming of motor patterns, and the second introduces a mark (German: *Zug*). This trait or mark (with Ernst: oh and ah) merely indicates that (an intangible) something is or remains exactly a Thing to the extent that it *cannot* be grasped or understood by a motor program. Phonemic and articulated signifiers, although written down, remain symbolic. Indeed, they structurally overshoot or fall short of the Thing.

This distinction between grasping or comprehending and marking or symbolising clarifies the repetition compulsion as endless attempts at the level of marking/symbolising that are, however, structurally disconnected from actual gratification. According to Bazan, the initial helplessness of the human child combined with the subtleties of symbolic language[25] differentiates humans from other animals. The mental or verbal object looms out of the missed encounter with the Thing. It is a concave container that can never quite (grasp/comprehend) the Thing.[26] We strive for a final word, but we can never quite say all we need to say because something remains unsayable or unwritable.[27] As with any coin, there is a brighter flip side. After all, without the endless repetition compulsion that drives this endeavour, there would be no culture, art, science, poetry, prose or... (neuro-) psychoanalysis.[28] Like Franz Schubert's symphony, they are all and necessarily *Unvollendet*, for the '*sapere*' or thinking of homo sapiens paradoxically owes its (continued) existence to its failure! In this context, I am reminded of a saying by the novelist Haruki Murakami[29]: 'The moment feelings are expressed in words, they turn into lies'.

And as for the signifier. While I was writing this final, another monthly column by Ariane Bazan appeared in one of our best Belgian dailies. It was entitled *De Naam van de Matroos* (The Name of the Sailor).[30] I transpose her thesis, with some simplification, into English. When people are first shown a print of the sun and of a scooter (which is called a 'step' in Dutch) and are then asked what they think of when they hear the word 'family', they answer 'step son' statistically significantly more often than other possibilities. Bazan's conclusion: phonology and not semantics work decisively here. Indeed, her column relies on a large-scale empirical study (n = 1468) that illustrates how the imprints of a rebus induce words in the subjects' unconscious that make their mark further down the line. She comments for a more general readership on the effect of the phonetic (rather than the semantic) of language and meanings on us. Thus, we *think* the images of the world around us directly fuel their meanings. In doing so, we regard language (only) as a *tool* for expression and communication. Yet, it seems that (unasked for and unknowingly) the things around us also trigger their associations *themselves*. In dreams and jokes, we can appreciate or even laugh at/enjoy this play of the signifier. And although it is beyond our scope, our daily functioning is also riddled with it.

That this sounds crazy or unreasonable may be evident from the disbelief and unpleasure (if not hilarity) often aroused by such (typically Lacanian) approaches. There is the risk, moreover, of the impression being created that psychoanalysis is (purely) a game of language and jousting, when, of course, it is above all about our affective lives that we (try to) process and edit in words and images. The neocortical cloak installed upon our limbic system and brain stem creates a buzz of algorithms running outside our awareness. They are linguistic in a digital way, and they originate from the big Other by whom we are surrounded from the start.[31]

That is why I will conclude with my prologue's two giants of psychoanalysis. Jacques Lacan recounts how Sigmund Freud – standing on the deck as he entered New York Harbour – turned to his pupil Carl Gustav Jung with the words: 'They don't realise we're bringing them the plague'.[32] To Lacan, it is not just about the plague of psychoanalysis but, more generally, the plague of the unconscious and of language. We are both scarred and plagued by both. They turn the human condition into fantastic misery.

Endnotes

1 Bazan and Detandt (2017, p. 2). In particular, I quote verbatim: 'From a mental perspective, we have proposed that Lacan's theory deploys a logical order to situate the repetition compulsion (Bazan and Detandt 2013). This temporal logic would involve (1) the emerging drive, (2) an experience of satisfaction, (3) accumulating bodily tension (upon reminiscing stimuli) and finally, (4) a repetition compulsion. Moreover, we have proposed that these four logical times found equivalence in different aspects of the mesolimbic dopaminergic system, namely (1) Panksepp's seeking system (Panksepp 1998); (2) Schultz's reward dopamine spike (Schultz 1998); (3) Olds and Milner's "pleasure" centre (Olds and Milner 1954); and (4) Berridge and Robinson's incentive sensitisation' (ibid.).
2 Schönau (2002).
3 I reiterate earlier thoughts on this (Kinet 2006b, 2013).
4 Stern (1985).
5 Stern et al. (1998).
6 Pope (1970 [1711]).
7 Eliot (2004 [1951]).
8 De Roder (1999).
9 Between mother and child and between loved ones, pet names carrying a private emotional charge and history are exchanged. A similar vocabulary is also formed between the poet and muse.
10 Lacan (1986) *La sublimation élève l'objet à la dignité de la Chose*. Sublimation elevates the object to the dignity of the Thing.
11 Van Ostaijen (1979). He (1896–1928) is the most influential poet Flanders has ever produced. Every avant-garde movement since the interwar years has drawn inspiration from his work, and at the same time, he has developed into the most enduringly popular modern Flemish poet.
12 Winnicott (1971, p. 17).
13 Van Ostaijen (1952) *Marc groet 's morgens de dingen*. See Dutch and English version https://www.poetryinternational.com/nl/poets-poems/poems/poem/103-6645_MARC-GREETS-THINGS-IN-THE-MORNING
14 Bazan (2016a), Bazan and Detandt (2015).
15 Freud (1895b).
16 Pickmann (2003, p. 41).
17 For recent discussions on trauma, see Kinet (2016a, 2016b). In my interlude 'Infinitely Less than Zero', I talked about zero-process thinking (petrification) versus the '*infinity*' of the unconscious.
18 Freud (1914a, p. 288, 1914b, p. 150).
19 Lacan (1973, p. 26).
20 Schultz (1998), Bazan (2016a), Bazan and Detandt (2013, 2015).
21 Robinson and Berridge (2000).

22 Lacan (1973, p. 51).
23 Hebbrecht (2010). I explained that Paul Verhaeghe (2002) distinguished actual pathology and psychopathology. In the former, raw and undigested drive and trauma exert their disruptive effect on psychological and physical functioning. In the latter, this is where a symptom's (linguistically structured) envelope has formed. Peter Fonagy (Fonagy and Target 2003) introduced a similar difference between mental process disorders and mental representational disorders. In the former, insufficient mental metabolisation takes place; in the latter, it is not processes but rather mental contents (and their mutual conflicts) that are problematic. Especially in the case of actual pathology and mental process disorders, therapy aims at subject-amplification and mentalising. They increase the affect-and-drive regulation and the possibility of trauma processing. In other words, psychopathology involves the more classic conflict neuroses, with their proliferation of the symbolic-imaginary that needs to be deconstructed and analysed. Actual pathology requires the construction and mental elaboration of structural (drive) and accidental trauma (Verhaeghe 1998). In Dutch and in German, there is respectively 'grijpen en begrijpen'/'greifen und begreifen'. To grasp an object but also to grasp a meaning.
24 I take my inspiration to simplify from a (for psychoanalytic insiders) *must-read* by Van De Vijver, Bazan, and Detandt (2017).
25 With its (re-) combinable units coming from the (mirroring) small other and the (marking) big Other.
26 Of course, with words like container and grasping, I am deliberately bridging the gap to the symbolising alpha function that plays such a major role in the *theory of thinking* of the Bionians (Vermote 2018).
27 Lacan (1973) draws inspiration from Aristotle in his distinction between different causalities: the necessary, the accidental/contingent and the impossible. The necessary is the *automaton* as that which does not cease to write itself (*ce qui ne cesse pas de s'écrire*). It is repetition at the level of signifiers. It is lawful. The accidental/contingent is what ceases not to write itself (*ce qui cesse de ne pas s'écrire*). It is the *tuchè* or chance: unpredictable. The third category is the impossible as the real that by definition is not symbolisable. It is what does not cease *not* to write itself (*ce qui ne cesse pas de ne pas s'écrire*).
28 Van de Vijver, Bazan, and Detandt (2017, p. 9).
29 Murakami (2011, p. 78).
30 When subjects are shown first a print of a 'matte' (Dutch: '*mat*') and then of a rose ('*roos*') and they are asked about their first association with the word 'ship' ('*schip*'), they are statistically significantly more likely to answer 'sailor' ('*matroos*'). To Bazan, this is a convincing (experimental) indication that the signifier inhabits and defines our psyche in its phonetic (rather than semantic) capacity.
31 A clinical example. One patient, parentified by her hysterical and promiscuous mother, says she feels like a piece of meat 'on the grill': stuck and completely curled up. I ask her: grill with single l or double l (in Dutch, *grill* with a single l means: whim). Next, follows a whole chain of associations related to the insecurity and developmental arrest that her mother's unpredictable and infantile behaviour has caused in her. This moment in her psychoanalytic process engendered relevant material. Still, it is ephemeral compared to the working through and internalisation within a therapeutic encounter/relationship that went on for years. A more personal example: in the hey-days of my Oedipal period Martin ('I Have a Dream') Luther King was murdered and around the same time John Fitzgerald Kennedy became president of the United States and was subsequently murdered. My father's full name is Jan Franciscus Kinet. I dwelt on the initials MK and JFK, on the similarity of Kinet and Kennedy and most of all, I was very upset by these assassinations. In this example, the symbolic (of phonetics) and the imaginary meet.
32 Lacan (1955a, p. 336).

Chapter 20

Interlude
From Shorthand to Liquid Crystal Display

My mother was a bank clerk, and my father was an Air Force adjutant. They gave me a typical, vintage (Golden Fifties) upbringing. In elementary school, they had me trained in shorthand and touch-typing. Their premise was that whatever becomes of you later, these skills will always be to your benefit – agreed, although that could not be said of learning to play the melodica or various Orff instruments. Indeed, I found joy in hammering on a discarded Olivetti from my mother's office! Impressed by my hyperkinetic speed, I was thoroughly carried away in four languages.

Thanks to the advent of the computer, touch-typing has done me great favours. In team meetings, I lightly caress the keyboard with both hands, and in my imagination, I underscore the affects in or hidden between the lines, like a piano player. Shorthand also served me well in many classes and lectures (less and less frequently attended). Now, in the age of YouTube and podcasts, I have once again dusted off some old faithful shorthand characters, which provide me with a great wealth of quotes and one-liners. I use them abundantly because what better tool is there to open heavily armed doors?

Metaphorically, shorthand also comes in handy. Take, for example, the most common feelings in our daily lives. To find a man or woman attractive is simply an evolutionarily efficient way of assessing their adaptive advantage. Beauty provides quick information: jawline and shoulder width indicate men's testosterone levels, whereas waist-to-hip ratio or full lips are visual expressions of women's oestrogen levels. Feelings, then, can be considered a shorthand of evolution: a brief and convenient representation of something that could be expressed in a much more complex way (by using language, for example).

Back to touch-typing. Sometimes my Ipad suddenly and inexplicably changes from an AZERTY to a QWERTY keyboard. Only after pressing the character 'a' several times (and producing the character 'q') do I realise something is wrong. The same stimulus leads to a different signifier, for what are the a and q other than phonetic and motor-articulated elements that acquire their meaning only within their context?

DOI: 10.4324/9781003394358-20

There is an error that forces me to abandon my automatism and to have another, broader and deeper look. This seems an excellent metaphor for Freud's false cross-linking (*falsche Verknüpfung*) or what current neuroscience says occurs in reconsolidation. The error message makes the screen of my consciousness flash on, and only then does it become apparent which program is running silently and where it needs updating or correction. As James Joyce put it: mistakes are the portals of discovery. Neuropsychoanalyst Mark Solms calls this consciousness by surprise. It is only when we falter or stumble that we learn from experience. Otherwise, we carry on as we are (for better or worse).

Through Solms, I can create a bridge between the Id and the unconscious or between his neuropsychoanalysis and Jacques Lacan. To do this, I must advance a few decades to the era of the liquid crystal display. At the beginning of our lives, we find ourselves in the proto-mental. It is the primordial soup about which French-speaking Bionians speak of the baby swimming in *O/le bébé qui nage dans l'O*. From the beginning, there is *logos* (mistranslated as in the beginning was the word because what is meant is the reason), and we formed concepts and hypotheses. In that sense, we were all once (for the proverbial fifteen minutes of fame) the greatest theorist on earth.

Probably chaos turns into cosmos, as in the book of Genesis, distinguishing between light and darkness (of presence and absence), pleasure and unpleasure. The unconscious can arise through repression as soon as the infant can express thoughts in language. To the Lacanians, there are no meanings in the unconscious, only signifiers. The letter is the smallest combinable part, which is why the initials that appear in *Mmmmama* and *Pppapa* are so important. However nonsensical, MK played a leading role in my former preference for Melanie Klein and Milan Kundera. It was their initiative *and* their initials that I identified with.

Repression buries the signifier but not the affect slipping and sliding through consciousness. To Solms, consciousness *is* affect, and the latter is the subjective and phenomenal sensation of the drives and instincts of the Id. The orphaned affect wanders the psyche in search of another signifier to which it can attach itself. However, the 'choice' of this signifier is not accidental but determined by the laws/*automaton* of the signifying chain. Displacement/metonymy and condensation/metaphor are the basic principles there.

Lionel Bailly[1] uses a wonderful and fitting image in his introduction to Jacques Lacan. Albeit that the confusion between the Id and the unconscious persists. He describes the unconscious (this should be the Id because the unconscious is a memory system and the Id a drive system) as a force field orienting the molecules in the liquid crystal display. The signifiers form connections under the influence of a hidden energy source. The Id speaks/*ça parle*. It is the thinking thing, the unconscious subject or the subject of the unconscious. It pushes or shoves signifiers forward. Also, or not in the least, a signifier that had been repressed.

Like a ball that, after being pushed underwater, follows its erratic course to the surface, it suddenly emerges as if out of nowhere. The surface of the water is like the silver screen of a cinema on which projection both from the inside and the outside world occurs. It acts as an interface. It teems with signifiers coming from the big Other, some of which, like paint, take to the wood of drive and affect. They bind free energy. Or not.

Endnote

1 Bailly (2009).

Chapter 21

Epilogue

In my previous publications, I have repeatedly defended a distinctly integrative position.[1] This position is sometimes confused with a more superficial eclecticism or pluralism. Still, to the contrary, it is characterised by a solid Freudian strain that can accommodate many branches (and even exotic grafts). Depending on the perspective used, the human/psychic comprises numerous elements that always foreground or highlight different aspects. The view of the drive had fallen into disuse, and the Ego, the object, the self, mentalisation or attachment successively took the upper hand within a psychoanalytic movement that, after Freud's *Big Bang,* has not only expanded but has also drifted apart. This is why I referred to Freud's premise at the beginning of this book: any progress is only half as big as it appears initially.[2]

Conversely, the therapeutic relationship is the womb (Latin: *matrix*) of the psychoanalytic process. Within it, too, the pursuit of integration is central.[3] Integration between conscious, pre-conscious and unconscious, between Id, Ego and Super-ego, between split-off or dissociated contents or processes or between different perspectives on what takes place within the encounters according to the patient and according to the moment.

On the one hand, neuropsychoanalysis provides little new for clinical practice. It would be best to look not to researchers but to thoroughbred clinicians for clinical nuances. However, it often confirms what had already been distilled from experience from a different angle. From an empirical angle, for example, neuropsychoanalysis demonstrates the need for sufficiently prolonged and intensive treatment. Both consolidation and reconsolidation, learning and unlearning, require neuroses to repeat and repeat a lot. Transference is a ubiquitous prediction error that, as such, must be interpreted, exposed and replaced by more realistic and up-to-date experiences.

Metapsychological speculations about drive, dreams, psychic energy and the successive models of our mind can also be correlated with neuroscientific findings and sometimes corrected or finetuned by them. If the clinical situation is hypothesis-generating, empirical-scientific research can (help to) confirm it. This strengthens the position of a psychoanalysis that is cherished almost as a creed[4] by its insiders but that has been relegated to a pseudo-scientific doom by the wider academic, scientific and social world.

DOI: 10.4324/9781003394358-21

Man has much more in common with animals than he has long wanted to acknowledge or accept. However, this can by no means be called a fault. Animals live in a biotope, and man within a horizon. The animal lives in a natural environment, but man breaks out of this seclusion and creates a world. Both utopia and dystopia are among his possibilities.[5] We are – as Nietzsche noted – sick animals. Our art, religion, science and technology can sweeten the pill, but it is increasingly questionable whether they transcend palliative care's impact.

I hope that both the more or less psychoanalytically initiated and the critical intellectual has found sufficient inspiration in this book. What does it conclude? The spirit of the drive is of immense affective-existential and evolutionary significance. After taking a poetic licence, I will allow myself another poetic hyperbole: neuropsychoanalysis may be the *nuclear physics* of our emotional life.

Endnotes

1 I work on this in almost all of my publications, but I refer in particular to my clinical psychotherapy triptych on (semi-)residential psychoanalytic hospitalisation-based treatment for (posttraumatic and other) anxiety, mood and personality disordered patients (2006, 2018, 2021). A translated and elaborated version of the first book is forthcoming: Psychoanalytic Principles in Psychiatric Practice: A Remedy by Truth (Routledge, accepted).
2 Freud (1926a, p. 286; 1926b, p. 175).
3 Strive for integration because, of course, this is a point beyond the horizon and therefore, by definition, a *mission impossible*.
4 In which various gospels are subjected to exegesis in 'catacombs'.
5 Gray (2014, p. 163): 'There may be a sense in which other animals are poor, but their poverty is an ideal that humans will never attain'. See also his article on Freud as the last great Enlightenment thinker (Gray, 2012).

References

Abraham, K. (1988 [1907]) The experiencing of sexual traumas as a form of sexual activity. In: K. Abraham (Ed.), *Selected Papers on Psychoanalysis*. London: Karnac: 47–62.

Ackrill, J. L. (1994) *Aristoteles*. Groningen: Historische Uitgeverij.

Aguiar, A. (2018) The 'real without law' in psychoanalysis and neurosciences. *Frontiers in Psychology*, 9: 851. https://doi.org/10:3389/fpsyg:2018:00851.

Alcaro, A., Carta, S., & Panksepp, J. (2017) The affective core of the self: A neuro-archetypical perspective on the foundations of human (and animal) subjectivity. *Frontiers in Psychology*, 8, Article 1424. https://doi.org/10.3389/fpsyg.2017.01424

Alisobhani, A., & Corstorphine, G. (2019) *Explorations in Bion's 'O'*. London/New York: Routledge.

Andreasen, N., O'Leary, D. S., Cizadlo, T. e.a. (1995) Remembering the past: Two facets of episodic memory explored with positron emission tomography. *American Journal of Psychiatry*, 152: 1576–1585.

Andrews-Hanna, J. R., Reidler, J. S., Huang, C., & Buckner, R. L. (2010) Evidence for the default network's role in spontaneous cognition. *Journal of neurophysiology*, 104(1): 322–335.

Ansermet, F., & Magistretti, P. (2004) *A chacun son cerveau. Plasticité neuronale et inconscient*. Paris: Odile Jacob.

Ansermet, F., & Magistretti, P. (2007) *Biology of freedom: Neural plasticity, experience, and the unconscious* (S. Fairfield, Trans.). New York: Other Press.

Anzieu, D. (1975) *L'auto-analyse de Freud — et la découverte de la psychanalyse*. Paris: PUF.

Anzieu, D. (1985) *Le moi-peau*. Paris: Dunod.

Arendt, H. (1998 [1958]) *The human condition*. Chicago: University of Chicago Press.

Ashby, W. R. (1962) *Principles of self-organizations: Transaction*. New York: Pergamon Press.

Aulagnier, P. (2003) *La violence de l'interprétation: du pictogramme à l'énoncé*. Paris: PUF.

Baars, B. J. (2003a) The fundamental role of context: Unconscious shaping of conscious information. In: B. J. Baars, W. P. Banks & J. B. Newman (Eds.) *Essential sources in the scientific study of consciousness*. Cambridge: MIT Press: 761–775.

Baars, B. J. (2003b) How does a serial, integrated, and very limited stream of consciousness emerge from a nervous system that is mostly unconscious, distributed, parallel and of enormous capacity? In: B. J. Baars, W. P. Banks & J. B. Newman (Eds.) *Essential sources in the scientific study of consciousness*. Cambridge: MIT Press: 1123–1129.

Bacon, F. (2000 [1620]) *The New Organon* (L. Jardine & M. Silverthorn, Eds.) New York: Cambridge University Press.

Badiou, A. (1988) *L'Etre et l'événément*. Paris: Du Seuil.

Bailly, L. (2009) *Lacan: A beginners guide*. London: One World Publications.

Balchin, R., Barry, V., Bazan, A., Blechner, M. J., Clarici, A., Mosri, D. F., Fotopoulou, A., Goergen, M. S., Kessler, R., Matthis, I., Zúñiga, J. F. M., Northoff, G., Olds, D., Oppenheim, L., Reismann-Lagrèze, D., Tsakiris, M., Watt, D., Yeates, G., & Zellner, M. (2019) Reflections on 20 years of Neuropsychoanalysis. *Neuropsychoanalysis*, 21(2): 89–123.

Balint, M. (1992 [1968]) *The basic fault. Therapeutic aspects of depression*. London: Tavistock.

Balkt, ter H. H. (2000) *Waterwingebieden* [Water catchment areas]. Amsterdam: De Bezige Bij.

Bargh, J. A., & Chartrand, T. L. (1999) The unbearable automaticity of being. *American Psychologist*, 54(7): 462.

Bateson, G. (2002 [1979]) *Mind and nature: A necessary unity*. London: Hampton Press.

Baudelaire, C. (1876) *Les Fleurs du Mal*. Paris: Larousse, 2011.

Bazan, A. (2002) The unconscious as affect sticking to phonology: Considerations on the role of articulation. *Psychoanalytische Perspectieven*, 20(4): 579–590.

Bazan, A. (2005) La forme du langage en clinique. Une perspective neuropsychanalytique. *Psychologie Clinique*, 18: 51-97.

Bazan, A. (2006) Primary process language. *Neuro-Psychoanalysis*, 8(2): 157–159.

Bazan, A. (2007a) *Des fantômes dans la voix. Une hypothèse neuropsychanalytique sur la structure de l'inconscient*. Collection Voix Psychanalytiques. Montréal: Editions Liber.

Bazan, A. (2007b) An attempt towards an integrative comparison of psychoanalytical and sensorimotor control theories of action. In: P. Haggard, Y. Rossetti, & M. Kawato (Eds.) *Attention and performance XXII*. New York: Oxford University Press: 319–338.

Bazan, A. (2009) Not to be confused on free association. *Neuropsychoanalysis*, 11: 163–165.

Bazan, A. (2010) Betekenaars in hersenweefsel: Bijdrage tot een fysiologie van het on-bewuste. In: [Signifiers in brain tissue: contribution to a physiology of the unconscious] Mark Kinet & Ariane Bazan (Eds.) *Psychoanalyse en Neurowetenschap: De geest in de machine* [Psychoanalysis and neuroscience: The ghost in the machine]. Antwerpen/Apeldoorn: Garant: 29–57.

Bazan, A. (2011a) The grand challenge for psychoanalysis – and neuropsychoanalysis: Taking on the game. *Frontiers in Psychology*, 2: 220.

Bazan, A. (2011b) Phantoms in the voice: A neuropsychoanalytic hypothesis on the structure of the unconscious. *Neuro-Psychoanalysis*, 13(2): 161–176.

Bazan, A. (2012) From sensorimotor inhibition to Freudian repression: Insights from psychosis applied to neurosis. *Frontiers in Psychology*, 3: 452.

Bazan, A. (2013) Repression as the condition for consciousness. Invited commentary on: "The conscious Id", M. Solms. *Neuropsychoanalysis*, 25(1): 20–24.

Bazan, A. (2014a) Neuropsychoanalyse: geschiedenis en epistemologie [Neuropsychoanal-ysis: history and epistemology]. *Tijdschrift voor Psychoanalyse*, 4: 245–255.

Bazan, A. (2014b) Waarom verdringen het soort vergeten is dat bewust maakt. Voorstel voor een breinmechanisme [Why repression is a kind of forgetting that renders con-scious. Proposition for a brain mechanism]. In: Marc Hebbrecht & Lili Philippe (Eds.) *Van verdringen tot vergeten. Een psychoanalytische herwerking van het geheugen* [From repression to forgetting. A psychoanalytic elaboration of memory]. Antwerpen/Apeldoorn: Garant: 21–44.

Bazan, A. (2015) Het wezenlijke van seks. Een metapsychologische denkoefening op het snijvlak tussen neurowetenschap en psychoanalyse [The essence of sex. A metapsychological exercise of thought on the border between neuroscience and psychoanalysis]. In: M. Kinet & K. Baeten (Eds.) *Psychoanalyse en/als seksuologie?* [Psychoanalysis and/as Sexology]. Antwerpen/Apeldoorn: Garant: 37–59.

Bazan, A. (2016a) Trauma en de Dopaminerge Inschrijving van het Evenement. Aan Gene Zijde van het Lustprincipe ligt de Demonische Herhalingsdwang [Trauma and the dopaminergic inscription of the event. Beyond the Pleasure Principle lies the demonic repetition compulsion]. In: Mark Kinet (Ed.) *Trauma binnenstebuiten* [Trauma inside out]. Antwerpen/Apeldoorn: Garant: 95–116.

Bazan, A. (2016b) Epistemologisch dualisme en de subversie van het Body-Mind vraagstuk: hoe psychoanalyse helpt het brein te ontcijferen [Epistemological dualis mand the subversion of the body-mind question: how psychoanalysis helps to decipher the brain]. In: M. Kinet & M. Thys (Eds.) *Psychoanalytische praktijk tussen onbewuste en wetenschap* [The practice of psychoanalysis between unconscious and science]. Antwerpen/Apeldoorn: Garant: 57–80.

Bazan, A. (2017) Alpha synchronization as a brain model for unconscious defense: An overview of the work of Howard Shevrin and his team. *The International Journal of Psychoanalysis*, 98: 1443–1473. https://doi.org/10.1111/1745-8315.12629.

Bazan, A. (2018) Psychoanalysis and academia: Psychoanalysis at the crossroads between exact and human sciences. *International Forum of Psychoanalysis*, 27: 90–97. https://doi.org/10.1080/0803706X.2017.1392040.

Bazan, A., & Detandt, S. (2013) On the physiology of jouissance: Interpreting the mesolimbic dopaminergic reward functions from a psychoanalytic perspective. *Frontiers in Human Neuroscience*. https://doi.org/10.3389/fnhum.2013.00709

Bazan, A., & Detandt, S. (2015) Trauma and jouissance, a neuropsychoanalytic perspective. *Journal of the Centre for Freudian Analysis and Research* (JCFAR), 26: 99–127.

Bazan, A., & Detandt, S. (2017) The grand challenge for psychoanalysis and neuropsychoanalysis: A science of the subject. *Frontiers in Psychology*, 8: 1259. https://doi.org/10.3389/fpsyg.2017.01259.

Beck, M. (2010) Beside Freud's Couch, a Chow named Jofi. *Wall Street Journal* (21/12/2010).

Belzen, Van J. A. (1988) *Fenomenologie en Psychiatrie. Essays van H.C. Rümke* [Phenomenology and Psychiatry]. Kampen: KokAgora.

Berridge, K. C. (1996) Food reward: Brain substrates of wanting and liking. *Neuroscience and Biobehavioral Reviews,* 20: 1–25. https://doi.org/10.1016/0149-7634(95)00033-B.

Berridge, K. C. (1999) Pleasure, pain, desire and dread: Hidden core processes of emotion. In: D. Kahneman, E. Diener, & N. Schwarz (Eds.) *Well being: The foundations of hedonic psychology*. New York: Russell Sage Foundation: 527–559.

Berridge, K. C. (2007) The debate over dopamine's role in reward: The case of incentive salience. *Psychopharmacology*, 191: 391–431. https://doi.org/10.1007/s00213-006-0578-x.

Berridge, K. C. (2009) "Liking" and "wanting" food rewards: Brain substrates and roles in eating disorders. *Physiology & Behavior*, 97(5): 537–550.

Berridge, K. C., & Kringelbach, M. L. (2008) Affective neuroscience of pleasure: Reward in humans and animals. *Psychopharmacology*, 199: 457–480. https://doi.org/10.1007/s00213-008-1099-6.

Bion, W. R. (1962) *Learning from experience*. London: Heinemann.

Bion, W. R. (1992) *Cogitations*. London/New York: Routledge.

Blass, R. B., & Carmeli, Z. (2007) The case against neuropsychoanalysis. On fallacies underlying psychoanalysis' latest scientific trend and its negative impact on psychoanalytic discourse. *International Journal of Psychoanalysis*, 88: 19–40.

Blass, R., & Carmeli, Z. (2015) Further evidence for the case against neuropsychoanalysis: How Yovell, Solms, and Fotopoulou's response to our critique confirms the irrelevance and harmfulness to psychoanalysis of the contemporary neuroscientific trend. *International Journal of Psychoanalysis*, 96: 1555–1573.

Bloom, P. (2013) *Just babies: The origins of good and evil*. New York: Crown.

Boer, Den J. A. (2003) *Neurofilosofie – hersenen, bewustzijn, vrije wil* [Neurophilosophy – brain, consciousness, free will]. Amsterdam: Boom.

Boer, Den J. A., & Glas, G. (2005) Over hersenen en mentale processen: theorie en conceptuele problemen [On the brain and mental processes: Theory and conceptual problems]. In: Jos De Kroon (Red.) *Hoe wetenschappelijk is de psychiatrie?* [How scientific is psychiatry?]. Antwerpen/Apeldoorn: Garant: 9–48.

Bollas, C (1987) *The shadow of the object: Psychoanalysis of the unthought known*. New York: Columbia University Press.

Boszormenyi-Nagy, I., & Spark, G. M. (1984) *Invisible loyalties: Reciprocity in intergenerational family therapy*. New York: Brunner/Mazel.

Bowen-Moore, P. (1989) *Hannah Arendt's philosophy of natality*. London: Macmillan.

Bowlby, J. (1969) *Attachment and loss: Vol I. Attachment*. New York: Basic Books.

Bowlby, J. (1973) *Attachment and loss: Vol II. Separation*. New York: Basic Books.

Bowlby, J. (1988) *A secure base. Clinical applications of attachment theory*. London: Routledge.

Bradley, M. M., & Lang, P. J. (1994) Measuring emotion: The self-assessment manikin and the semantic differential. *Journal of Behavior Therapy and Experimental Psychiatry*, 25(1): 49–59.

Bradshaw, G. A., Schore, A.N., Brown, J. L. Poole, J. H., & Moss, C. J. (2005) Elephant breakdown. Social trauma: Early disruption of attachment can affect the physiology, behavior and culture of animals and humans over generations. *Nature*, 2005(433): 807.

Bremner, J. D. (1999) Does stress damage the brain? *Biological Psychiatry*, 1999(45): 797–805.

Brenner, C. (1982) *The mind in conflict*. New York: International Universities Press.

Bucci, W. (1997) *Psychoanalysis and cognitive science: A multiple code theory*. New York: Guilford.

Buckner, R. L., Andrews-Hanna, J. R., & Schacter, D. L. (2008) The brain's default network: Anatomy, function, and relevance to disease. *Annals of the New York Academy of Sciences*, 1124(1): 1–38.

Burgdorf, J., & Panksepp, J. (2006) The neurobiology of positive emotions. *Neuroscience & Biobehavioral Reviews*, 30(2): 173–187.

Campbell, W. K., & Sedikides, C. (1999) Self-threat magnifies the self-serving bias: A meta-analytic integration. *Review of general Psychology*, 3(1): 23–43.

Carhart-Harris, R., & Friston, K. (2010) The default-mode, ego-functions and free-energy: A neurobiological account of Freudian ideas. *Brain*, 133: 1265–1283.

Carhart-Harris, R. L., & Friston, K. J. (2012) Free-energy and Freud: An update. In: A. Fotopoulou, D. W. Pfaff, & E. M. Conway (Eds.) *Trends in neuropsychoanalysis: Psychology, psychoanalysis and cognitive neuroscience in dialogue*. Oxford: Oxford University Press: 219–229.

Castanet, H. (2022) *Neurologie versus psychanalyse*. Paris: Navarin.

Chalmers, D. (1995a) Facing up to the problem of consciousness. *Journal of Consciousness Studies*, 2: 200–219.

Chalmers, D. (1995b) *The conscious mind: In search of a fundamental theory*. New York: Oxford University Press.

Chalmers, D. (2022) *Human brains: It begins with an idea*. Venezia: Fondazione Prada.

Changeux, J. P. (1983) *L'homme neuronal*. Paris: Fayard.

Char, R. (1983) Œuvres complètes. Paris: Gallimard, coll. Bibliothèque de la Pléiade.

Churchill, W. (2001) *The wicked wit of Winston Churchill*. London: Michael O'Mara books.

Churchland, P. (2022) *Human brains: It begins with an idea*. Venezia: Fondazione Prada.

Ciano, Di P., Cardinal, R. N., Cowell, R. A., Little, S. J., and Everitt, B. J. (2001) Differential involve-ment of NMDA, AMPA/kainate, and dopa- mine receptors in the 14 nucleus ac-cumbens core in the acquisition and performance of pavlovian approach behavior. *Journal of Neuroscience*, 21: 9471–9477.

Cioran, E. (1988) *Aveux et anathèmes*. Paris: Gallimard.

Clark, A. (2016) *Surfing uncertainty: Prediction, action and the embodied mind*. London: Oxford University Press.

Cluckers, G. & Meurs, M. (2005) Bruggen tussen denk-wijzen [Bridges between ways of thinking]. In: Mark Kinet en Rudi Vermote (Red.) *Mentalisatie*. Antwerpen/Apeldoorn: Garant: 11–34

Clyman, R. B. (1991) The procedural organization of emotions – A contribution from cogni-tive science to the psychoanalytic theory of therapeutic action. *Journal of the American Psychoanalytic Association*, 39, Suppl: 349–382.

Coillie, Van F. (2022) Het probleem van de seksualiteit. Wat is het probleem? [The problem of sexuality. What is the problem?]. *Tijdschrift voor Psychoanalyse & haar toepassingen*, 4: 254–264.

Colace, C. (2012) Dream bizarreness and the controversy between the neurobiological ap-proach and the disguise-censorship model: The contribution of children's dreams. *Neu-ropsychoanalysis*, 14: 165–174.

Coleridge, S. T. (2004 [1816]) *Christabel, Kubla Khan, and the Pains of Sleep*. In: W. Keach (Ed.) *The Complete Poems*. London/New York: Penguin Books: 55–58

Collingwood, R. G. (2005 [1933]) *An essay on philosophical method* (James Connelly & Giuseppina D'Oro, Eds.). Oxford: Oxford University Press.

Cook, V., & Newson, M. (2014) *Chomsky's universal grammar: An introduction*. London/New York: Wiley.

Crane, T., & Patterson, S. (2001) *History of the mind-body problem*. London/New York: Routledge, 2001.

Crick, F. (1995 [1994]) *Astonishing hypothesis: The scientific search for the soul*. London: Scribner

Damasio, A. (2014 [1994]) *Descartes' error: Emotion, reason and the human brain*. New York: Random House.

Damasio, A. (2000 [1999]) *The feeling of what happens: Body and emotion in the making of consciousness*. London: Mariner Books.

Damasio, A. (2010) *Het gelijk van Spinoza. Vreugde, verdriet en het voelende brein* [Look-ing for Spinoza. Joy, sorrow and the feeling brain]. Amsterdam: Wereldbibliotheek.

Damasio, A. (2021 [2018]) *The strange order of things: Life, feeling and the making of cultures*. London: Robinson.

Darwin, C. (2003 [1859]) *The origin of species*. London/New York: Signet, 2003.

Darwin, C. (1981 [1871]) *The descent of man and selection in relation to sex. (facsimile)*. Princeton: Princeton University Press, 1981.

Darwin, C. (2009 [1872]) *The expression of emotions in man and animals*. London/New York: Penguin.

Davies, M. (2010) Double dissociation: Understanding its role in cognitive neuropsychology. *Mind & Language*, 25(5) November 2010: 500–540.

Dawkins, R. (1996) *The blind watchmaker: Why the evidence of evolution reveals a universe without design*. London/New York: Norton & Company.

Declercq, F. (2000) *Het Reële bij Lacan* [The real in Lacan]. Gent: Idesça.

Deleuze, G. (2003) *Spinoza: Philosophie pratique*. Paris: Minuit.

Derrida, J. (1980) *Pour l'amour de Lacan*. Paris: Flammarion

Derrida, J. (1988) *Limited Inc*. Evanston: Northwestern University Press.

Diamond, N. (2013) *Between skins: The body in psychoanalysis – contemporary developments*. Chichester: John Wiley & Sons.

Dijksterhuis, A. P. (2008) *Het slimme onbewuste* [The smart unconscious]. Amsterdam: Prometheus.

Dilthey, W. (1988 [1883]) *Introduction to the human sciences: An attempt to lay a foundation for the study of society and history*. Detroit: Wayne State University Press.

Dirkx, J (2016) Van psychoanalyse naar neuroanalyse. Is er een alternatief? [From psychoanalysis to neuroanalysis. Is there an alternative?]. *Tijdschrift voor Psychoanalyse*, 4: 256–268.

Doidge, N. (2007) *The brain that changes itself*. New York: Viking.

Draaisma, D. (2010) *Vergeetboek; wat we over vergeten moeten weten* [The book of forgetting. What we have to know about forgetting]. Groningen: Historische Uitgeverij.

Du Bois-Reymond, E. (1918) *Letter to Hallmann, 1842. Jugendbriefe von Emil Du Bois-Reymond an Eduard Hallmann*. Berlin: Dietrich Reimer.

Dunn, J. (2003) Have we changed our view of the unconscious in contemporary clinical work? *Journal of the American Psychoanalytic Association*, 51: 941–955.

Eagle, M. N. (2011) *From classical to contemporary psychoanalysis: A critique and integration*. London/New York: Routledge.

Eichenbaum, H. (1998) Amnesia, the hippocampus and episodic memory. *Hippocampus*, 1998(8): 97.

Eichenbaum, H. (1999) Conscious awareness, memory and the hippocampus. *Nature Neuroscience*, 2(9): 775–776.

Ekman, P. (2013 [1972]) *Emotion in the human face*. Los Altos: Malor Books.

Eliot, T. S. (2001 [1922]) *The waste land*. New York: W.W.Norton: 1–20.

Eliot, T. S. (1998 [1920]) Hamlet and his problems. In: *The sacred wood and major early essays*. New York: Dover: 55–59.

Ellis, G., & Solms, M. (2018) *Beyond evolutionary psychology: How and why neuropsychological modules arise*. Cambridge: Cambridge University Press.

Emde, R. (1991) Positive emotions for psychoanalytic theory: Surprises from infancy research and new directions. In: T. Shapiro & R. Emde (Ed.) *Affect: Psychoanalytic perspectives*. Madison: International Universities Press: 5–44.

Engel, G. (1962) *Psychological development in health and disease*. Philadelphia: Saunders.

Erickson, M. (1992) *Onbewust leren* [Unconscious learning]. Drempt: Uitgeverij Karnak.

Etchegoyen, R. H. (1999) *The fundamentals of psychoanalytic technique.* London/New York: Karnac Books, 2nd Edition.

Etchegoyen, R. H., & Miller, J. A. (1996) *Silence Brisé. Entretien sur le mouvement psychanalytique.* Paris: Agalma Diffusion Seuil.

Etkin, A., Phil, M., Pittinger, C., Polan, H. J., & Kandel, E. R. (2005) Toward a neurobiology of psychotherapy: Basic science and clinical applications. *The Journal of Neuropsychiatry and Clinical Neurosciences,* 17(2): 145–158. http://dx.doi.org/10.1176/jnp.17.2.145. PMID: 15939967

Evans, D. (1996) *An introductory dictionary of Lacanian psychoanalysis.* London: Routledge.

Ferenczi, S. (1982 [1933]) Confusion de langue entre l'enfant et les adultes. *Psychanalyse* IV. Paris: Payot: 125–138.

Fernando, J. (2018) Trauma and the Zero Process: Clinical illustrations. *Psychoanalysis,* 29(3): 37–45.

Ferro, A., & Civitarese, G. (2015) *The psychoanalytic Field and its Transformations.* London/New York: Routledge.

Feynman, R. (2019) *What I cannot create, I do not understand. Richard Feynman Physics Notebook.* London: Quality Notebooks.

Feys, E. L. (2009) *L'anthropopsychiatrie de Jacques Schotte. Une introduction.* Paris: Editions Hermann.

Fink, B. (1997) *A clinical introduction to Lacanian psychoanalysis.* London: Harvard University Press.

Fisher, M. (2009) *Capitalist realism: Is there no alternative?* Winchester; Washington, DC: Zero Press.

Florio, M, Albert, M., Taverna, E., Namba, T., Brandl, T., e.a. (2015) Human-specific gene ARHGAP11B promotes basal progenitor amplification and neocortex expansion. *Science,* 347: 1465–1470.

Fonagy, P. (1999) Memory and therapeutic action. *International Journal of Psychoanalysis,* 80: 215–234.

Fonagy, P. (2003a) Genetics, developmental psychopathology, and psychoanalytic theory: The case for ending our (not so) splendid isolation. *Psychoanalytic Inquiry,* 23: 218–247.

Fonagy, P. (2003b) The interpersonal interpretive mechanism: The confluence of fentecis and attachment theory in development. In: V. Green (Ed.) *Emotional development in psychoanalysis, attachment theory and neuroscience: Creating connections.* New York: Brunner-Routledge: 107–126.

Fonagy, P. (2008) A genuinely developmental theory of sexual enjoyment and its implications for psychoanalytic technique. *The Journal of the American Psychoanalytic Association,* 56: 11–36.

Fonagy, P., & Target, M. (2018 [1998]) An interpersonal view of the infant. In: A. Hurry (Ed.) *Psychoanalysis and developmental therapy.* London: Routledge: 3–31

Fonagy, P., & Target, M. (2003) Fonagy and Target's model of mentalisation. In: A. Hurry (Ed.) *Psychoanalysis and developmental therapy.* London: Whurr: 270–282.

Fonagy, P., Gergely, G., Jurist, E. L., & Target, M. (2004) Affect regulation, mentalization, and the development of the self. Londen/New York: Karnac.

Fotopoulou, A., & Tsakiris, M. (2017) Mentalizing homeostasis: The social origins of interoceptive inference, *Neuropsychoanalysis,* 19(1): 3–28.

Freud, A. (1992[1936]) *The Ego and the mechanisms of defence*. London: The Institute of Psychoanalysis.

Freud, M. (1973) Freud: My father. In: H. M. Ruitenbeck (Ed.) *Freud as we knew him*. Detroit: Wayne State University Press: 180–185

Freud, S. (1892–1899) Extracts from the Fliess papers. In: J. Strachey (Ed.) *Standard edition of the complete psychological works of Sigmund Freud, 1*. London: Hogarth: 174–280.

Freud, S. (1893) Some points for a comparative study of organic and hysterical motor paralyses. In: J. Strachey (Ed.) *Standard edition of the complete psychological works of Sigmund Freud, 1*. London: Hogarth: 155–172.

Freud, S. (1894) The neuropsychoses of defence. In: J. Strachey (Ed.) *Standard edition of the complete psychological works of Sigmund Freud, 3*. London: Hogarth: 45–61.

Freud, S. (1895) Studies on hysteria. In: J. Strachey (Ed.) *Standard edition of the complete psychological works of Sigmund Freud, 2*. London: Hogarth: 1–321

Freud, S. (1895a) Extracts from the Fliess papers. In: J. Strachey (Ed.) *Standard edition of the complete psychological works of Sigmund Freud, 1*. London: Hogarth: 177–280.

Freud, S. (1895b) Project for a scientific psychology. In: J. Strachey (Ed.) *Standard edition of the complete psychological works of Sigmund Freud, 1*. London: Hogarth: 283–397.

Freud, S. (2006 [1900a]) De droomduiding. In: W. Oranje (Ed.) *Sigmund Freud Werken* 2. Amsterdam: Boom: 30–582.

Freud, S. (1900b) The interpretation of dreams. In: J. Strachey (Ed.) *Standard edition of the complete psychological works of Sigmund Freud, 4-5*. London: Hogarth: 339–627.

Freud, S. (2006 [1905a]) Drie verhandelingen over de theorie van de seksualiteit. In: W. Oranje (Ed.) *Sigmund Freud Werken 4*. Amsterdam: Boom: 15–116.

Freud, S. (1905b) Three essays on the theory of sexuality. In: J. Strachey (Ed.) *Standard edition of the complete psychological works of Sigmund Freud, 7*. London: Hogarth: 130–243.

Freud, S. (2006 [1909a]) Opmerkingen over een geval van dwangneurose [De 'Rattenman']. In: W. Oranje (Ed.) *Sigmund Freud Werken 5*. Amsterdam: Boom: 14–82.

Freud, S. (1909b) Notes upon a case of obsessional neurosis. In: J. Strachey (Ed.) *Standard edition of the complete psychological works of Sigmund Freud, 10*. London: Hogarth: 153–318.

Freud, S. (2006 [1911a]) Formuleringen over de twee principes van het psychische gebeuren. In: W. Oranje (Ed.) *Sigmund Freud Werken 5*. Amsterdam: Boom: 332–339.

Freud, S. (1911b) Formulations on the two principles of mental functioning. In: J. Strachey (Ed.) *Standard edition of the complete psychological works of Sigmund Freud, 12*. London: Hogarth: 218–226.

Freud, S. (1912) A note on the unconscious in psychoanalysis. In: J. Strachey (Ed.) *Standard edition of the complete psychological works of Sigmund Freud, 12*. London: Hogarth: 255–266.

Freud, S. (2006 [1912–1913a]) Totem en taboe. In: W. Oranje (Ed.) *Sigmund Freud Werken* 6. Amsterdam: Boom: 18–166.

Freud, S. (1912–1913b) Totem and taboo: Some points of agreement between the mental lives and savages and neurotics. In: J. Strachey (Ed.) *Standard edition of the complete psychological works of Sigmund Freud, 13*. London: Hogarth: 1–161.

Freud, S. (2006 [1913a]) Het belang bij de psychoanalyse. In: W. Oranje (Ed.) *Sigmund Freud Werken 6*. Amsterdam: Boom: 255–279.

Freud, S. (1913b) The claims of psychoanalysis to scientific interest. In: J. Strachey (Ed.) *Standard edition of the complete psychological works of Sigmund Freud, 13.* London: Hogarth: 165–190.

Freud, S. (2006 [1914a]) Herinneren, herhalen en doorwerken. In: W. Oranje (Ed.) *Sigmund Freud Werken.* Amsterdam: Boom: 287–294.

Freud, S. (1914b) Remembering, repeating and working through. In: J. Strachey (Ed.) *Standard edition of the complete psychological works of Sigmund Freud, 2.* London: Hogarth: 146–156.

Freud, S. (2006 [1915a]) De verdringing. In: W. Oranje (Ed.) *Sigmund Freud Werken 7.* Amsterdam: Boom: 45–60.

Freud, S.(1915b) Repression. In: J. Strachey (Ed.) *Standard edition of the complete psychological works of Sigmund Freud, 14.* London: Hogarth: 141–158.

Freud, S. (2006 [1915c]) Het onbewuste. In: W. Oranje (Ed.) *Sigmund Freud Werken 7.* Amsterdam: Boom: 65–102.

Freud, S. (1915d) The unconscious. In: J. Strachey (Ed.) *Standard edition of the complete psychological works of Sigmund Freud, 14.* London: Hogarth: 159–215.

Freud, S. (2006 [1915e]) Driften en hun lotgevallen. In: W. Oranje (Ed.) *Sigmund Freud Werken 7.* Amsterdam: Boom: 17–44.

Freud, S. (1915f) Instincts and their vicissitudes. In: J. Strachey (Ed.) *Standard edition of the complete psychological works of Sigmund Freud, 14.* London: Hogarth: 117–140.

Freud S (1917) A difficulty in the path of psycho-analysis. In: J. Strachey (Ed.) *Standard edition of the complete psychological works of Sigmund Freud 17.* London: Hogarth: 135–144.

Freud, S. (1920a) Aan gene zijde van het lustprincipe. In: W. Oranje (Ed.) *Sigmund Freud Werken 8.* Amsterdam: Boom: 162–218.

Freud, S. (1920b) Beyond the pleasure principle. In: J. Strachey (Ed.) *Standard edition of the complete psychological works of Sigmund Freud, 18.* London: Hogarth: 1–64.

Freud, S. (2006 [1921c]) Massapsychologie en Ik-analyse. In: W. Oranje (Ed.) *Sigmund Freud Werken 8.* Amsterdam: Boom: 225–292.

Freud, S. (1921d) Mass psychology and the analysis of the Ego. In: J. Strachey (Ed.) *Standard edition of the complete psychological works of Sigmund Freud, 18.* London: Hogarth: 69–143.

Freud, S. (2006 [1923a]) Het Ik en het Es. In: W. Oranje (Ed.) *Sigmund Freud Werken 8.* Amsterdam: Boom: 380–420.

Freud, S. (1923b) The ego and the id. In: J. Strachey (Ed.) *Standard edition of the complete psychological works of Sigmund Freud, 19.* London: Hogarth: 12–59.

Freud, S. (2006 [1926a]) Remming, symptoom en angst. In: W. Oranje (Ed.) *Sigmund Freud Werken 9.* Amsterdam: Boom: 186–286.

Freud, S. (1926b) Inhibitions, symptoms and anxiety. In: J. Strachey (Ed.) *Standard edition of the complete psychological works of Sigmund Freud, 14.* London: Hogarth: 77–175.

Freud, S. (2006 [1926c]) Het vraagstuk van de lekenanalyse. In: W. Oranje (Ed.) *Sigmund Freud Werken 9.* Amsterdam: Boom: 276-338.

Freud, S. (1926d) The question of lay analysis. In: J. Strachey (Ed.) *Standard edition of the complete psychological works of Sigmund Freud, 20.* London: Hogarth: 179–250.

Freud, S. (1930) Civilization and its discontents. In: J. Strachey (Ed.) *Standard edition of the complete psychological works of Sigmund Freud, 21.* London: Hogarth: 64–145.

Freud, S. (2006 [1933a]) Colleges inleiding tot de psychoanalyse. Nieuwe reeks. In: W. Oranje (Ed.) *Sigmund Freud Werken 10*. Amsterdam: Boom: 77–232.

Freud, S. (1933b) New introductory lectures on psycho-analysis. In: J. Strachey (Ed.) *Standard edition of the complete psychological works of Sigmund Freud 22*. London: Hogarth: 5–182.

Freud, S. (2006 [1940a]) Hoofdlijnen van de psychoanalyse. In: W. Oranje (Ed.) *Sigmund Freud Werken 10*. Amsterdam: Boom: 443–503.

Freud, S. (1940b) An outline of psychoanalysis. In: J. Strachey (Ed.) *Standard edition of the complete psychological works of Sigmund Freud, 23*. London: Hogarth: 144–207.

Freud, S. (1950) *The origins of psycho-analysis*. New York: Basic Books.

Freud, S. (1961) *Letters of Sigmund Freud 1873–1939* (Ernst L. Freud, Ed.; Tania and James Stern, Trans.). London: Hogarth.

Freud, S. (2006) Register van citaten en allusies [Register of quotes and allusions]. In: *Sigmund Freud Werken 11*. Amsterdam: Boom: 424–473.

Friston, K (2010) The free-energy principle: A unified brain theory? *Nature Reviews Neuroscience*, 11: 127–138.

Friston, K. (2013) Life as we know it. *Journal of the Royal Society*, 10: 20130475. http://dx.doi.org/10.1098/rsif.2013.0475

Fuchs, T. (2004) Neurobiology and psychotherapy: An emerging dialogue. *Current Opinion in Psychiatry*, 2004(17): 479–485.

Gaulejac, de V. (2013) Entre l'individu et le sujet, il y a toute une histoire ... Pour une approche socio-clinique des récits de vie. *Les Politiques Sociales*, 1–2: 108–120.

Glas, G. (2006) Ambiguïteit in Eric Kandel's neurowetenschappelijke fundering van de psychiatrie [Ambiguity in Eric Kandel's neuroscientific fundamentals of psychiatry]. *Tijdschrift voor Psychiatrie*, 48: 849–856.

Goethe, Von J. W. (1999 [1819]) *West-östlicher Divan*. Reclam: Frankfurt am Main.

Goldapple, K., Segal, Z., Garson, C., Lau, M., Bieling, P., Kennedy, S., & Mayberg, H. (2004) Modulation of cortical-limbic pathways in major depression: Treatment-specific effects of cognitive behavior therapy. *Archives of General Psychiatry*, 61: 34–41.

Goodall, J. (1986) *The chimpanzees of Gombe: Patterns of behavior*. Cambridge: Belknap Press.

Gould, S. J. (1981) *The mismeasure of man*. New York: Norton.

Gracian, B. (1647) *Handorakel* [Hand Oracle]. Amsterdam: Atheneum, 2016.

Gray, J. (2012) *Freud: The last great Enlightenment thinker*. https://www.prospectmagazine.co.uk/magazine/freud-the-last-great-enlightenment-thinker

Gray, J. (2014) *The silence of animals: On progress and other modern myths*. London: Farrar, Strauss & Giroux.

Green, A. (1995) *La causalité psychique entre nature et culture*. Paris: Odile Jacob.

Grinker, R. (2001) My father's Analysis with Sigmund Freud. *Annual of Psychoanalysis*, 29: 35–47.

Groddeck, G. (1977) *The meaning of illness: Selected psychoanalytic writings* (G. Mander, Trans.). London/New York: International Universities Press.

Grünbaum, A. (1984) *The foundations of psychoanalysis: A philosophical critique*. Berkeley: California University Press.

Haraway, D. (2015) Anthropocene, capitalocene, plantationocene, Chthulucene: Making kin. *Environmental Humanities*, 6: 159–165.

Hartmann, H. (1951) Ego psychology and the problem of adaptation. In: D. Rapaport (Ed.) *Organization and pathology of thought: Selected sources*. New York: Columbia University Press: 362–396. https://doi.org/10.1037/10584-019

Haute, Van P. (1990) *Het imaginaire en het symbolische in het werk van Jacques Lacan* [The imaginary and the symbolic in the work of Jacques Lacan]. Leuven: Peeters.

Haute, Van P. (2000) *Tegen de aanpassing* [Against adaptation]. Nijmegen: SUN.

Hebb, D. (2002 [1949]) *The organization of behavior*. New York: Lawrence Erlbaum.

Hebbrecht, M. (2010) *De droom. Verkenning van een grensgebied* [The dream: Exploration of a border territory]. Utrecht: De Tijdstroom.

Herman, J. L., Perry, J. C., & Kolk, B. A. van der. (1989) Childhood trauma in borderline personality disorder. *American Journal of Psychiatry*, 147: 490–495.

Hobson, J. A., & McCarley, R. W. (1977) The brain as a dream state generator: An activation-synthesis hypothesis of the dream process. *American Journal of Psychiatry*, 134: 1335–1348.

Hoorde, Van H. (2010) *Psychiatrie & Psychoanalyse. Een volgehouden dialoog* [Psychiatry and psychoanalysis: A sustained dialogue]. Gent: Academia Press.

Hume, D. ([2003] 1739) *A treatise of human nature*. London: Courier Corporation.

Jablonka, E., & Lamb, M. J. (2014) *Evolution in four dimensions, revised edition: Genetic, epigenetic, behavioral, and symbolic variation in the history of life*. Cambridge: MIT Press.

Jackson, F. (2002 [1986]) What Mary didn't know. In: P. K. Moser and J. D. Trout (Eds.) *Contemporary materialism*. London/New York: Routledge: 198–202.

Jaspers, K. (1913) *Algemeine Psychopathologie*. Berlin: Springer.

Johnson, B. (2008) Just what lies beyond the pleasure principle? *Neuropsychoanalysis*, 10: 201–212.

Johnson, B., & Flores Mosri, D. (2016) The neuropsychoanalytic approach: Using neuroscience as the basic science of psychoanalysis. *Frontiers in Psychology*, 7(1459): 2–12.

Johnston, A. (2013) Drive between brain and subject: An immanent critique of Lacanian neuropsychoanalysis. *The Southern Journal of Philosophy*, 51: 48–84.

Joyce, J. (2012 [1922]) *Ulysses*. London: Oxford University Press.

Joyce, J. (2020 [1939]) *Finnegans wake*. London/New York: Penguin Classics.

Kandel, E. R. (1998) A new intellectual framework for psychiatry. *American Journal of Psychiatry*, 155: 457–469.

Kandel, E. R. (1999) Biology and the future of psychoanalysis. *American Journal of Psychiatry*, 156: 505–524.

Kandel, E. R. (2006) *In search of memory*. New York: Norton.

Kandel, E. R. (2012) *The age of insight: The quest to understand the unconscious in art, mind, and brain, from Vienna 1900 to the present*. New York: Random House.

Kaplan-Solms, K., & Solms, M. (2000) *Clinical studies in neuro-psychoanalysis: Introduction to a depth psychology*. London: Karnac.

Kapuszinsky, R. (2006) *De Ander. Essays van de reporter van de eeuw* [The other. Essays from the reporter of the century]. Amsterdam/Antwerpen: Arbeiderspers.

Kenny, D. T. (2013) *Bringing up baby: The psychoanalytic infant comes of age*. London: Karnac Books.

Kenny, D. T. (2019) Faulty theory, failed therapy: Frances Tustin, infant and child psychoanalysis, and the treatment of autism spectrum disorders. SAGE Open, 9(1): 2158244019832686.

Kernberg, O. F. (1975) *Borderline states and pathological narcissism*. New York: Jason Aronson.

Kernberg, O. F. (1976) *Object relations theory and clinical psychoanalysis*. New York: Jason Aronson.

Kesel, De M. (2005) Een sociomaterieel psyche [A sociomaterial psyche]. In: Jos De Kroon (Red.) *Hoe wetenschappelijk is de psychiatrie?* [How scientific is psychiatry?]. Antwerpen/Apeldoorn: Garant: 111–128.

Kesel, De M. (2009) *Het münchausenparadigma. Waarom Freud en Lacan ertoe doen* [The münchhausen paradigm. Why Freud and Lacan matter]. Nijmegen: Van Tilt.

Kihlstrom, J. F. (1996) Perception without awareness of what is perceived, learning without awareness of what is learned. In: M. Velmans (Ed.) *The Science of Consciousness: Psychological, Neuropsychological, and Clinical Reviews*: London: Routledge: 23–46. https://doi.org/10.4324/9780203360019_chapter_2

Killeen, P. R. (2003) Complex dynamic processes in sign tracking with an omission contingency (negative automaintenance). *Journal of Experimental Psychology*, 29(1): 49–61.

Kinet, M. (1992) Clinical psychotherapy and acting-out. http://www.markkinet.be/pdf/009%20Clinical%20psychotherapy%20and%20acting-out.pdf

Kinet, M. (1996) Weerzien met … Melanie Klein [Melanie Klein revisited]. *Tijdschrift voor Psychotherapie*, 3: 197–211.

Kinet, M. (2002) Het passieprincipe: NoThing but the Real Thing [The passion principle: noThing but the Real Thing] In: Mark Kinet & Michel Thys (Red.) *Liefdesverklaringen. Over perversie, liefde en passie* [Love Statements. On perversion, love and passion]. Leuven/Leusden: Acco: 155–177.

Kinet, M. (2005) Reflections in a golden I. In: M. Kinet & L. Moyson (Red.) *Grootse patiënten, kleine therapeuten. Narcisme en psychotherapie* [Grand patients, small therapists. Narcissism and psychotherapy]. Antwerpen/Apeldoorn: Garant: 7–19.

Kinet, M. (2006a) *Freud & co in de psychiatrie. Klinisch-psychotherapeutisch perspectief* [Freud & co in psychiatry. A clinical psychotherapy perspective]. Antwerpen/Apeldoorn: Garant.

Kinet, M. (2006b) Poëzie en psychoanalyse, muze en mentalisatie [Poetry and psychoanalysis, muse and mentalisation] In: M. Kinet & R. Vermote (Red.) *Mentalisatie*. Antwerpen/Apeldoorn: Garant: 111–128.

Kinet, M. (2008a) Lacaniaanse neuropsychoanalyse. *Tijdschrift voor Psychoanalyse*, 4: 285–287.

Kinet, M. (2008b) Empathie en empathologie. Als het register van het imaginaire [Empathy and empathology as the order of the imaginary] In: Marc Hebbrecht en Ingrid Demuynck (Red.) *Empathie in psychoanalytische psychotherapie* [Empathy in psychoanalytic psychotherapy] Antwerpen/Apeldoorn: Garant: 101–115.

Kinet, M. (2009a) Psychoanalyse van en in de groep. Van ideologie tot subject [Psychoanalysis of and in the group. From ideology to subject] In: M. Kinet (Red.) *De groep in psychoanalyse* [The group in psychoanalysis]. Antwerpen/Apeldoorn: Garant: 11–32.

Kinet, M. (2009b) Over een kader dat geen passe-partout is [On a frame that is not a passe-partout]. *Tijdschrift Klinische Psychologie*, 39(2): 90–98.

Kinet, M. (ed.) (2010a) *Parentificatie. Als het kind te snel ouder wordt* [Parentification. When the child ages too fast]. Antwerp/Apeldoorn: Garant.

Kinet, M. (2010b) Van neuronen en neurosen. fMRI van de ziel [On neurons and neuroses. fMRI of the soul] In: M. Kinet & A. Bazan (Red.) *Psychoanalyse en neurowetenschap. De geest in de machine* [Psychoanalysis and Neuroscience. The Ghost in the Machine]. Antwerpen/Apeldoorn: Garant: 79–110.

Kinet, M. (2010c) A cry in the dark. Appel en antwoord in psychoanalytisch perspectief [A cry in the dark. Appeal and answer in a psychoanalytic perspective]. In: W. Roelofsen e.a.

(Red.) *Psychoanalytische Psychotherapie over Grenzen* [On the boundaries of Psychoanalytic Psychotherapy]. Assen: Van Gorcum: 41–50.

Kinet, M. (2011a) Elvis van de psychoanalyse. [Elvis of psychoanalysis]. *Tijdschrift voor Psychoanalyse* (2): 135–136.

Kinet, M (2011b) Obiit Joyce McDougall (1920–2011) *Tijdschrift voor Psychoanalyse*, 4: 42–43.

Kinet, M. (2013b) De vierkantswortel van super. Supervisie vanuit klinisch psychotherapeutisch perspectief. [The square root of super. Supervision in a clinical psychotherapy perspective]. In: M. Hebbrecht, N. Vliegen (Red.) *Supervisie. Van psychoanalyse en psychoanalytische therapie*. Antwerpen/Apeldoorn: Garant: 123–140.Kinet, M. (2015a) Spreekt het lichaam (de waarheid)? [Does the body speak (the truth)?] In: Mark Kinet, Katrien Vuylsteke-Vanfleteren, Sjef Houppermans (Red.) *Als het lichaam spreekt* [When the body speaks]. Antwerpen/Apeldoorn: Garant: 7–20.

Kinet, M. (2015b) Tussen diepte- en metaseksuologie. Psychoanalyse met het Es van seks [Between depth- and metasexuology. Psychoanalysis with the Es of Sex] In: M. Kinet & K. Baeten (Red.) *Psychoanalyse als seksuologie?* [Psychoanalysis as sexology]. Antwerpen/Apeldoorn: Garant: 61–86.

Kinet, M. (2015d) Karl Abraham 1877–1925. Freud's rots in de branding [Karl Abraham. Freud's Rock Solid]. *Tijdschrift voor Psychiatrie*, (4): 294–295. https://www.tijdschriftvoorpsychiatrie.nl/nl/artikelen/article/50-10532_Karl-Abraham-1877-1925-Freuds-rots-in-de-branding

Kinet, M. (Red.) (2016a) *Trauma binnenstebuiten. Verbanden bij psychische wonden* [Trauma inside out]. Antwerpen/Apeldoorn: Garant.

Kinet, M. (2016b) Het trauma als zwart gat. Van metastasen tot permanente catastrofe. In: [Trauma as a black hole. From metastases to permanent catastrophe] M. Kinet (Red.) *Trauma binnenstebuiten* [Trauma inside out]. Antwerpen/Apeldoorn: Garant: 71–94.

Kinet, M. (2017) *Onderzocht en ondervonden. Over de wetten van de passies* [Examined and experienced: on the laws of the passions]. Antwerpen/Apeldoorn: Garant.

Kinet, M. (2018) *Een psychotherapeutische praktijk. In 7 premissen en 77 portretten* [A psychotherapy practice in 7 premises and 77 portraits]. Oud-Turnhout/'s Hertogenbosch: Gompel-Svacina.

Kinet, M. (2019) Enkele oedipale variaties. Van Darwin tot Lacan [Some oedipal variations. From Darwin to Lacan]. In: M. Kinet & W. Heuves (Red.) *Driehoeksverhoudingen Actuele oedipale variaties* [Triangles. Current oedipal variations]. Hertogenbosch: Gompel & Svacina: 51–70.

Kinet, M. (2020) Psychoanalytische geestigheden [Psychoanalytic Wit]. *Tijdschrift voor Psychoanalyse*, 2: 136–138.

Kinet, M. (2021a) *Beter en wijzer door psychotherapie. 31 patiënten vertellen het zelf* [Better and wiser through psychotherapy. 31 patients tell it themselves]'s. Hertogenbosch: Gompel & Svacina.

Kinet, M. (2021b) Het hondbewuste [Das Hundbewusste]. *Tijdschrift voor Psychoanalyse*, 1: 61–62.

Kinet, M. (2021c) Infinitely less than zero. *Tijdschrift voor Psychoanalyse*, 3: 212–214.

Kinet, M. (2022a) Psychoanalytische posologie [Psychoanalytic Posology]. *Tijdschrift voor Psychoanalyse*, 3: 194–196.

Kinet, M. (2022b) Kent & I. *Tijdschrift voor Psychoanalyse*, 1: 54–55.

Kinet, M. (2022c) De groep: het onbewuste live on stage [The group: the unconscious live on stage]. *Tijdschrift voor Groepsdynamica & Groepspsychotherapie*, 2: 24–41.

Kinet, M. (2022d) *De geest van de drift. Over neuropsychoanalyse*. Antwerpen/'s Hertogenbosch: Gompel & Svacina.

Kinet, M. (2023) Enkele voorlaatste woorden. Tussen ça voir en faire ainsi [A few penultimate thoughts. Between ça voir and faire ainsi]. In: M. Hebbrecht & C. Franckx (Eds.) *Het kinderlijk trauma. Verloren tussen tederheid en passie* [Childhood trauma. Lost between tenderness and passion]. Antwerpen/'s Hertogenbosch: Gompel & Svacina: 295–306.

Kinet, M., & Bazan, A. (Red.) (2010) *Psychoanalyse en neurowetenschap. De geest in de machine* [Psychoanalysis and Neuroscience. The Ghost in the Machine]. Antwerpen/Apeldoorn: Garant.

Kinet, M., & Heuves, W. (Red.) (2019) *Driehoeksverhoudingen. Actuele oedipale variaties* [Triangles. Current oedipal variations]. Antwerpen/'s Hertogenbosch: Gompel & Svacina.

Kirchhoff, M., Parr, T., Palacios, E., Friston, K., & Kiverstein, J. (2018) The Markov-blankets of life: Autonomy, active inference and the free energy principle. *Journal of the Royal Society Interface*, 15: 1–12.

Klein, M. (1957) Envy and gratitude. In: *The writings of Melanie Klein. (Vol IV)*. London: Hogarth Press: 180.

Kloet, De E. R. (2009) Stress: Neurobiologisch perspectief [Stress: neurobiological perspective]. *Tijdschrift voor Psychiatrie*, 8: 547.

Kloos, W. (2017 [1894]) *Verzen* [Verses]. Nijmegen: Van Tilt.

Koenig, J. (2022) *The dictionary of obscure sorrows*. New York: Simon & Schuster.

Kohn, E. (2013) *How forests think: Toward an anthropology beyond the human*. Oakland: University of California Press.

Kristeva, J. (1984) *Revolution in poetic language*. New York: Columbia University Press.

Kroon, De J. (2004) *Schizofrenie tussen symptoom en subject. Een archeologie van de psychose* [Schizophrenia between symptom and subject. An archaeology of psychosis]. Antwerpen/Apeldoorn: Garant.

Kroon, De J. (2005) *Hoe wetenschappelijk is de psychiatrie?* [How scientific is psychiatry?]. Antwerpen/Apeldoorn: Garant.

Krupenye, C., & Call, J. (2016) Theory of mind in animals: Current and future directions. *Wiley Interdisciplinary Reviews: Cognitive Science*, 10(6): e1503.

Kuyper, S. (1977) *Dagen uit het leven* [Days of life]. Amsterdam: De Bezige Bij.

LaBar, K. S., & Cabeza, R. (2006) Chronic stress hormones impair memory retrieval and hippocampal function as exemplified by PTSD (Cognitive neuroscience of emotional memory. *Nature Reviews Neuroscience*, 7: 54–64.

Lacan, J. (1949) Le stade du miroir comme formateur de la fonction du Je. In: J. Lacan (Ed.) *Ecrits*. Paris: Du Seuil: 93–100.

Lacan, J. (1950) Propos sur la causalité psychique. In: J. Lacan (Ed.) *Ecrits*. Paris: Du Seuil: 151–196.

Lacan, J. (1952) Intervention sur le transfert. In: J. Lacan (Ed.) *Ecrits*. Paris: Du Seuil: 215–228.

Lacan, J. (1953a) Fonction et champ de la parole et du langage en psychanalyse. In: J. Lacan (Ed.) *Ecrits*. Paris: Du Seuil: 237–322.

Lacan, J. (1953b) Le Symbolique, l'Imaginaire et le Réel. In: J. Lacan and J. A. Miller (Eds.) *Des Noms-Du-Père*. Paris: Du Seuil: 9–63.

Lacan, J. (1955a) Variantes de la cure-type. In: J. Lacan (Ed.) *Ecrits*. Paris: Du Seuil: 323–362.

Lacan, J. (1955b) La chose freudienne ou Sens du retour à Freud en psychanalyse. In: J. Lacan (Ed.) *Ecrits*. Paris: Du Seuil: 401–436.

Lacan, J. (1956) Le Séminaire sur 'la lettre volée'. In: J. Lacan (Ed.) *Ecrits*. Paris: Du Seuil: 11–61.

Lacan, J. (2006 [1957]) The instance of the letter in the unconscious or reason since Freud. In: J. Lacan & J. A. Miller (Eds.) *Ecrits*. New York: Norton: 412–442.

Lacan, J. (1958a) La direction de la cure et les principes de son pouvoir. In: J. Lacan (Ed.) *Ecrits*. Paris: Du Seuil: 585–645.

Lacan, J. (1958b) La signification de phallus. In: J. Lacan (Ed.) *Ecrits*. Paris: Du Seuil: 685–696.

Lacan, J. (1958c) La jeunesse de Gide ou la lettre et le désir. In: J. Lacan (Ed.) *Ecrits*. Paris: Du Seuil: 739–764.

Lacan, J. (1959) Sur la théorie du symbolisme d'Ernest Jones. In: J. Lacan (Ed.) *Ecrits*. Paris: Du Seuil: 697–717.

Lacan, J. (1960a) Remarque sur le rapport de Daniel Lagache : 'Psychanalyse et structure de personnalité. In: J. Lacan (Ed.) *Ecrits*. Paris: Du Seuil: 647–684.

Lacan, J. (1960b) Propos directifs pour un Congrès sur la sexualité féminine. In: J. Lacan (Ed.) *Ecrits*. Paris: Du Seuil: 725–738.

Lacan, J. (1962) Kant avec Sade. In: J. Lacan (Ed.) *Ecrits*. Paris: Du Seuil: 765–790.

Lacan, J. (1966) *Ecrits*. Paris: Du Seuil.

Lacan, J. (1966a) De nos antécédents. In: J. Lacan (Ed.) *Ecrits*. Paris: Du Seuil: 65–72.

Lacan, J. (1966b) La science et la vérité. In: J. Lacan (Ed.) *Ecrits*. Paris: Du Seuil: 855–877.

Lacan, J. (1973) *Le Séminaire. Livre XI. Les Quatre Concepts Fondamentaux de la Psychanalyse, 1963–1964* (J.-A. Miller, Ed.). Paris: Du Seuil.

Lacan, J. (1975a) *Le Séminaire. Livre I. Les écrits techniques de Freud. 1953–1954*. Texte établi par J. A. Miller. Paris: Du Seuil.

Lacan, J. (1975b) *Le Séminaire Livre XX. Encore. 1972–1973*. Texte établi par J. A. Miller. Paris: Du Seuil.

Lacan, J. (1981a) *Le Séminaire Livre III. Les psychoses. 1955–1956*. Texte établi par J. A. Miller. Paris: Du Seuil.

Lacan, J. (1981b) *The Seminar. Book XI, The Four Fundamental Concepts of Psychoanalysis, 1963–1964* (A. Sheridan, Trans.). New York: Norton.

Lacan, J. (1986) *Le Séminaire. Livre VII. L'éthique de la psychanalyse. 1959–1960*. Texte établi par J.A. Miller. Paris: Du Seuil.

Lacan, J. (1988b) *The Seminar. Book II. The Ego in Freud's theory and in the Technique of Psychoanalysis. 1954–1955*. Translated Sylvana Tomaselli, notes by John Forrester. New York: Norton.

Lacan, J. (1991a) *Le Séminaire. Livre VIII. Le transfert. 1960–1961*. Texte établi par J. A. Miller. Paris: Du Seuil.

Lacan, J. (1991b) *Le Séminaire. Livre XVII. L'envers de la psychanalyse. 1969–1970*. Texte établi par J.A. Miller. Paris: Du Seuil.

Lacan, J. (1992) *The Seminar. Book VII. The Ethics of Psychoanalysis. 1959–1960*. Translated Dennis Porter, notes by Dennis Porter. London: Routledge.

Lacan, J. (1994) *Le Séminaire Livre IV. La relation d'objet. 1956–1957*. Texte établi par J. A. Miller. Paris: Du Seuil.

Lacan, J. (1998) *Le Séminaire Livre V. Les formations de l'inconscient. 1957–1958*. Paris: Du Seuil.

Lacan, J. (2002) *The Seminar. Book IX. Identification. 1961–1962*. Cormac Gallagher. London: Karnac.

Lacan, J. (2005) *Le Séminaire Livre XXIII Le Sinthome. 1975–1976*. Texte établi par J. A. Miller. Paris: Du Seuil.

Lacan, J (2011a) Savoir, ignorance, verité et jouissance. *Je parle aux murs*. Paris: Du Seuil.

Lacan, J. (2017a) *Le Séminaire, Livre XIII: L'objet de la Psychanalyse 1965–1966*. Texte établi par J. A. Miller. Paris: Du Seuil.

Lacan, J. (2017b) *Le Séminaire Livre XIV La Logique du Fantasme, 1966–1967*. (M. Roussan, Ed.). Paris: Du Seuil.

Ladan, A. (2000) *Het wandelend hoofd. Over de geheime fantasie een uitzondering te zijn* [The walking head. On the secret phantasy of being an exception]. Amsterdam: Boom.

Ladan, A. (2006) Enkele opmerkingen over het geheugen [Some remarks on memory]. *Tijdschrift voor Psychoanalyse* 12(2): 194–201.

Langs, R. (1982) *Psychotherapy, a basic text*. New York/London: Jason Aronson.

Laplanche, J. & Pontalis, J. B. (1967) *Vocabulaire de la Psychanalyse*. Paris: Presse Universitarie de France.

Lauwaert, L (2021) *Wij, robots. Een filosofische blik op technologie en artificiële intelligentie* [We, robots. A philosophical view on technology and artificial intelligence]. Tielt: Lannoo Campus.

LeDoux, J. E. (1994) Emotion, memory and the brain. *Scientific American*, 6: 32–39.

LeDoux, J. E. (1996) *The emotional brain: The mysterious underpinnings of emotional life*. New York: Touchstone.

Leffert, M. (2010) *Contemporary psychoanalytic foundations. Postmodernism, complexity and neuroscience*. New York/London: Routledge.

Lichtenberg, J. D. (2013) Development and psychoanalysis: Then and now-the influence of infant studies. *Psychoanalytic Review*, 100(6): 861–880.

Liu, D., Diorio, J., Tannenbaum, B., Caldji, C., Francis, D., Freedman, A., Sharma, S., Pearson, D., Plotsky, P. M., & Meaney,M. J. (1997) Maternal care, hippocampal glucocorticoid receptors, and hypothalamic-pituitary-adrenal responses to stress. *Science, 277:* 1659–1662.

Lombardo, R., Rinaldi, L., & Thanopulos, S. (2019) *Psychoanalysis of the psychoses. Current developments in theory and practice*. London/New York: Routledge.

Luyten, P. (2019) Psychoanalyse en onderzoek: uit de «splendid isolation» [Psychoanalysis and research: Out of the splendid isolation]. *Tijdschrift voor Psychoanalyse*, 25(1): 5–16.

Luyten, P., Blatt, S. J., & Corveleyn, J. (2006) Minding the gap between positivism and hermeneutics in psychoanalytic research. *Journal of the American Psychoanalytic Association*, 54: 571–610.

MacLean, P. D. (1990) *The triune brain in evolution: Role in paleocerebral functions*. New York: Plenum Press.

Main, M., & Goldwyn, S. (1995) Interview based adult attachment classification: Related to infant-mother and infant-father attachment. *Developmental Psychology*, 19: 237–239.

Mancia, M. (2006) *Neuropsychoanalysis and neuroscience*. Milan: Springer Verlag.

Masson, J. M. (1985) *The complete letters of Sigmund Freud to Wilhelm Fliess, 1877–1904*. Cambridge: Harvard University Press.

Masson, O. (2019) *L'invention lacanienne : du retour à Freud (1951–1957) à la construction de l'objet a (1958–1963) Une archéologie critique de la pensée de Jacques Lacan*. Paris: Psychologie Université Paris Cité.

Matte-Blanco, I. (1988) *Thinking, feeling and being*. London/New York: Routledge.

Mayberg, H. (2007) Defining the neural circuitry of depression: Toward a new nosology with therapeutic implications. *Biological Psychiatry*, 61: 729–730.

McCabe, D., & Castel, A. (2008) Seeing is believing: The effect of brain images on judgments of scientific reasoning. *Cognition*, 107: 343–352.

McDougall, J. (1982) *Theatres of the body. A psychoanalytic approach to psychosomatic illness*. London: Free Association Books.

McWilliams, N. (2011) *Psychoanalytic diagnosis: Understanding personality structure in the clinical process*. New York: The Guilford Press.

Meaney, M. J. (2001) Maternal care, gene expression, and the transmission of individual differences in stress reactivity across generations. *Annual Review of Neuroscience*, 24: 1161–1192.

Merker, B. (2007) Consciousness without a cerebral cortex: A challenge for neuroscience and medicine. *Behavioral and Brain Sciences*, 30(1): 63–81.

Milner, J.-C. (2000) *De la linguistique à la linguisterie*. Paris: Flammarion.

Mooij, A. (2002) *Psychoanalytisch Gedachtegoed* [Psychoanalytic Thought]. Amsterdam: Boom.

Moruzzi, G., & Magoun, H. (1949) Brain stem reticular formation and activation of the EEG. *Electrocephalography and Clinical Neurophysiology*, 1(4): 455–473.

Mosri, D. F. (2021) Clinical applications of neuropsychoanalysis: Hypotheses toward an integrative model. *Frontiers in Psychology*. https://doi.org/10.3389/fpsyg.2021.718372

Mulisch, H. (2010) *De ontdekking van de hemel* [The discovery of heaven]. Amsterdam: Bezige Bij.

Murakami, H. (2011) *After the quake*. London/New York: Random House.

Nabokov, V. (1980) *Lectures on literature*. New York: Harcourt Brace Jovanovich.

Nader, K., Schafe, G. E., & LeDoux, J. E. (2000) The labile nature of consolidation theory. *Nature Reviews Neuroscience*, 1(3): 216–219.

Nagel, T. (1974) What is it like to be a bat? *The Philosophical Review*, 83(4): 435–450.

Nagel, T. (2012) *Mind and cosmos: Why the materialist neo-Darwinian conception of nature is almost certainly false*. Oxford: Oxford University Press.

Nasio, J.-D. (1992) *Cinq leçons sur la théorie de Jacques Lacan*. Paris: Rivages.

Nicolai, N. J. (2009) Chronische stress, sekse en gender [Chronic stress, sex and gender]. *Tijdschrift voor Psychiatrie*, 8: 569–577.

Nicolai, N. J. (2014) Van ratten en mensen. Jaak Panksepp en de affectieve neurowetenschap [Of rats and men. Jaak Panksepp and affective neuroscience]. *Tijdschrift voor Psychoanalyse*, 4: 277–284.

Nicolai, N. J. (2017) *Emotieregulatie als basis van het menselijk bestaan. De kunst van het evenwicht* [Emotion regulation at the base of human existence. The art of balance]. Leusden: Diagnosis.

Nietzsche, F. (1980 [1878]) *Menselijk, al te menselijk. Een boek voor vrije geesten* [Human, all too human]. Amsterdam: Synopsis.

Nietzsche, F. (2022 [1885]) *Aldus sprak Zarathustra* [Thus Spoke Zarathustra]. Amsterdam: Wereldbibliotheek.

Nietzsche, F. (2004 [1886]) *Voorbij goed en kwaad* [Beyond good and evil]. Amsterdam: Arbeiderspers.

Nieweg, E. H. (2005) 'De psychiater in spagaat: over de kloof tussen natuur- en geesteswetenschappen' [The split of the psychiatrist: On the gap between natural and human sciences]. *Tijdschrift voor Psychiatrie*, 47: 239–248.

Nobus, D. (1998) *Key concepts of Lacanian psychoanalysis*. London: Rebus Press.

Ogden, T. (1999) The music of what happens in poetry and psychoanalysis. *International Journal of Psychoanalysis*, 80: 979–994.

Ogden, T. (2004) The analytic third: Implications for psychoanalytic theory and technique. *The Psychoanalytic Quarterly*, 73(1): 167–195.

Olds, J., & Milner, P. (1954) Positive reinforcement produced by electrical stimulation of septal area and other regions of rat brain. *Journal of Comparative and Physiological Psychology*, 47: 419–427.

Olyff, G & Bazan, A (2023) People solve rebuses unwittingly—Both forward and backward: Empirical evidence for the mental effectiveness of the signifier. *Frontiers in Human Neuroscience*, 1–20 16: 965183. https://doi.org/10.3389/fnhum.2022.965183.

Ostaijen, Van P. (1996 [1952]) *Verzamelde gedichten* [Collected poems]. Amsterdam: Prometheus/Bert Bakker.

Ostaijen, Van P. (1979) *Gebruiksaanwijzing der lyriek* [User guide to lyricism]. *Verzameld werk/proza II.* Amsterdam: Bert Bakker.

Panksepp, J. (1971) Aggression elicited by electrical stimulation of the hypothalamus in albino rats. *Physiology & Behavior*, 6(4): 311–316.

Panksepp, J. (1998) *Affective neuro-science: The foundations of human and animal emotions.* New York: Oxford University Press.

Panksepp, J. (2007) Neuroevolutionary sources of laughter and social joy: Modelling primal human laughter in laboratory rats. *Behavioral Brain Research*, 182: 231–244.

Panksepp, J. (2011) Cross-species affective neuroscience decoding of the primal affective experiences of humans and related animals. *PloS One*, 6(9): e21236.

Panksepp, J., & Biven, L. (2012). *The archaeology of mind: Neuroevolutionary origins of human emotion.* New York Norton.

Panksepp, J., & Davis, K. (2018) *The emotional foundations of personality: A neurobiological and evolutionary approach.* New York: W. W. Norton & Company.

Panksepp, J., & Solms, M. (2012) What is neuropsychoanalysis? Clinically relevant studies of the minded brain. *Trends in cognitive sciences*, 16(1): 6–8.

Pastor, A. (2020) Memory systems of the brain. *arXiv preprint arXiv:2009.01083.*

Peirce, C. S. (1994) *Peirce on signs: Writings on semiotic* (James Hoopes, Ed.). Chapel Hill: University of North Carolina Press.

Peña-Guzmán, D. M. (2022) *When animals dream: The hidden world of animal consciousness.* New York: Princeton Press.

Penfield, W., & Boldrey, E. (1937) Somatic motor and sensory representation in the cerebral cortex of man as studied by electrical stimulation. *Brain*, 60(4): 389–443.

Perry, B. D. (2001) The neurodevelopmental impact of violence in childhood. In: D. Schetky & E. Benedek (Red.) *Textbook of child and adolescent forensic psychiatry.* Washington: American Psychiatric Press: 221–238.

Phillips, A (1988) *Winnicott.* Cambridge: Harvard University Press.

Phillips, A. (1994) *On flirtation.* Cambridge: Harvard University Press.

Phillips, A. (2014) *Freud. De geboorte van de psychoanalyticus* [Freud. The making of a psychoanalyst] Amsterdam: Ambo/Anthos.

Plant, D. (2012) A look at narcissism through Professor Higgins in Pygmalion. *British Journal of Psychotherapy*, 28(1): 50–65.

Pickmann, C. N. (2003) La rencontre traumatique du sexuel. *Figures de la psychanalyse*, 8(1): 41–49.

Pope, A. (1970 [1711]) *An essay on criticism.* Menston: Scolar Press.

Popper, K. (2014 [1963]) *Conjectures and refutations: The growth of scientific knowledge.* London/Routledge.

Porge, E. (1989) *Se compter trois. Le temps logique de Lacan.* Paris: Eres.

Ramachandran, V. S. (2003) *The emerging mind. BBC Reith Lectures 2003.* London: Profile Books.

Reekum, Van A., & Schmeets, M. (2008) De gen-omgevingsinteractie en de psychiatrie: nieuwe visie op de invloed van de vroege omgeving [Gen-environment interaction and psychiatry: a new vision of the influence of early environment]. *Tijdschrift voor Psychiatrie,* 12: 771–780.

Robinson, D. (1973) Twin masters: Pleasure and pain. In: D. Robinson (Ed.) *The Enlightened Machine: An Analytical Introduction to Neuropsychology.* New York Chichester, West Sussex: Columbia University Press: 119–134.

Robinson, T. E., & Berridge, K. C. (1993) The neural basis of drug craving: An incentive-sensitization theory of addiction. *Brain Research Reviews,* 18: 247–291.

Robinson, T. E., & Berridge, K. C. (2000) The psychology and neurobiology of addiction: An incentive-sensitization view. *Addiction* (Suppl.] 2): S91–S117.

Robinson, T. E., & Berridge, K. C. (2003) Addiction. *Annual Review of Psychology,* 54: 25–53.

Rocke, A. J. (2010) *Image and reality. Kekulé, Kopp and the scientific imagination.* Chicago: University of Chicago Press.

Roder, De J. H. (1999) *Het schandaal van de poëzie* [The scandal of poetry]. Nijmegen: Van Tilt.

Roffman, J. L., Marci, C. D., Glick, D. M., Dougherty, D. D., & Rauch, S. L. (2005) Neuroimaging and the functional neuroanatomy of psychotherapy. *Psychological Medicine,* 35: 1385–1398.

Roth, M. S. (2015) https://www.theatlantic.com/health/archive/2015/05/oliver-sacks-knows-what-it-really-means-to-live/393410/

Rothenberg, A. (1971) The process of Janusian thinking in creativity. *Archives of General Psychiatry* 24(3) (March 1): 195. https://doi.org/10.1001/archpsyc.1971.01750090001001.

Sacks, O. (1984) *A leg to stand on.* London: Duckworth.

Sacks, O. (1986) *The man who mistook his wife for a hat.* London: Duckworth.

Safouan, M. (2005) *Lacaniana. Les Séminaires de Jacques Lacan. 1964–1979.* Paris: Fayard.

Salas, C, Turnbull, O. & Solms, M. (2021) (Ed.) *Clinical studies in neuropsychoanalysis revisited.* London/New York: Routledge.

Sartre, J.-P. (1996 [1946]) *L'existentialisme est un humanisme.* Paris: Folio Essais.

Saussure, de F. (2002 [1916]) Écrits de linguistique générale (Simon Bouquet & Rudolf Engler, Eds.). Paris: Gallimard.

Schacter, D. L. (1996) *Searching for memory.* New York: Basic Books.

Schacter, D. L. (2001) *The seven sins of memory — How the mind forgets and remembers.* Boston/New York: Houghton Mifflin Company.

Schiller, D., Monfils, M., Raio, C. M., Johnson, D. C., LeDoux, J. E., & Phelps, E. A. (2010) Preventing the return of fear in humans using reconsolidation update mechanisms. *Nature,* 463: 49–53.

Schiller, F. (2016 [1794]) *On the aesthetic education of man*: London: Penguin Classics.

Schönau, W. (2002) De moeder-taal van de poëzie [The mother tongue of poetry]. In: *Psychoanalyse en poëzie* (Hillenaar en Nuyten, Red.). Amsterdam: Dutch University Press: 17–44.

Schore, A. N. (1994) *Affect regulation and the origin of the self: The neurobiology of emotional development.* Hilsdale: Lawrence Erlbaum Association.

Schore, A. N. (2003a) *Affect dysregulation and disorders of the self.* New York: Norton.

Schore, A. N. (2003b) *Affect regulation and the repair of the self.* New York: Norton.

Schotte, J. (2006) *Un parcours. Rencontrer, relier, dialoguer, partager.* Paris: Editions Le Pli.

Schultz, W. (1998) Predictive reward signal of dopamine neurons. *Journal of Neurophysiology,* 80: 1–27.

Searle, J. R. (1980) Minds, brains, and programs. *The Behavioral and Brain Sciences,* 3: 417–424.

Seminowicz, D. A., Mayberg, H. S., McIntosh, A. R., Goldapple, K., Kennedy, S. Segal, Z., & Rafi-Tari, S. (2004) Limbic-frontal circuitry in major depression: A path modeling metanalysis. *Neuroimage,* 22: 409–418.

Shakespeare, W. (1996 [1603–1604]) Hamlet. Prince of Denmark. In: *Complete Works.* London: Wordsworth: 670–713.

Shevrin, H. (1995) Is psychoanalysis one science, two sciences, or no science at all? A discourse among friendly antagonists. *Journal of the American Psychoanalytic Association,* 43: 963–986.

Shevrin, H. (2010) Een algemene psychoanalytische theorie verlaten. Wat zijn de gevolgen als we Rapaports poging in aanmerking nemen [Abandon a general psychoanalytic theory. What are the consequences taking into account Rapaport's effort]. In: Mark Kinet & Ariane Bazan (Red.) *Psychoanalyse en neurowetenschap. De geest in de machine.* Antwerpen-Apeldoorn: Garant: 11–28.

Shevrin, H., Bond, J. A., Brakel, L. A., Hertel, R. K., & Williams, W. J. (1996) *Conscious and unconscious processes: Psychodynamic, cognitive and neurophysiological convergences.* New York: Guilford Press.

Shevrin, H., Snodgrass, M., Brakel, L. A., Kushwaha, R., Kalaida, N. L., & Bazan, A. (2013) Subliminal unconscious conflict alpha power inhibits supraliminal conscious symptom experience. *Frontiers in Human Neuroscience,* 7: 544.

Sifneos, P. (1992) *Short-term anxiety-provoking psychotherapy: A treatment manual.* New York: Basic Books.

Silvio, J. R. (1985) George Bernard Shaw's Pygmalion: A creative response to early childhood loss. *Journal of the American Academy of Psychoanalysis,* 23(2): 234–243.

Sitskoorn, M. (2006) *Het maakbare brein* [The makeable brain]. Amsterdam: Bert Bakker.

Sitskoorn, M. (2010) *Passies van het brein. Waarom zondigen zo verleidelijk is* [Passions of the brain. Why it is so tempting to sin]. Amsterdam: Bert Bakker.

Siviy, S. M., & Panksepp, J. (2011) In search of the neurobiological substrates for social playfulness in mammalian brains. *Neuroscience & Biobehavioral Reviews,* 35(9): 1821–1830.

Skinner, B.F. (2005 [1953]) *Science and human behavior.* New York: MacMillan.

Solms, M. (1991) Summary and discussion of the paper 'The neuro psychological organisation of dreaming: implications for psychoanalysis'. *Bulletin of the Anna Freud Centre,* 16: 149–165.

Solms, M. (1997) *The neuropsychology of dreams: A clinico-anatomical study.* Mahwah: Lawrence Erlbaum Associates.

Solms, M. (1998) Before and after Freud's 'Project'. In R. Bilder & F. LeFever (Red.) *Neuroscience of the mind on the centennial of Freud's project for a scientific psychology. Annals of the New York Academy of sciences,* 843: 1-10.

Solms, M. (2000a) Dreaming and REM sleep are controlled by different brain mechanisms. *Behavioral and Brain Sciences*, 23: 843–850.

Solms, M. (2000b) Freud, Luria and the clinical method. *Psychoanalysis and History*, 2: 76–109.

Solms, M. (2001) The neurochemistry of dreaming: Cholinergic and dopaminergic hypotheses. In: E. Perry, H. Ashton & A. Young (Red.) *The Neurochemistry of Consciousness.* New York: John Benjamins: 123–131.

Solms, M. (2013a) The conscious id. *Neuropsychoanalysis*, 15: 5–19.

Solms, M. (2013b) Justifying psychoanalysis. *British Journal of Psychiatry*, 203: 389–391.

Solms, M. (2015a) Reconsolidation: Turning consciousness into memory. *Behavioral and Brain Sciences*, 38: 40–41.

Solms, M. (2015b) *The feeling brain: Selected papers on neuropsychoanalysis.* London: Karnac.

Solms, M. (2017a) Empathy and other minds – a neuropsychoanalytic perspective and a clinical vignette. In: V. Lux & S. Weigl (Red.) *Empathy: Epistemic problems and cultural-historical perspectives of a cross-disciplinary concept.* London: Palgrave Macmillan: 93–114.

Solms, M. (2017b) Consciousness by surprise: A neuropsychoanalytic approach to the hard problem. In: R. Poznanski, J. Tuszynski, & T. Feinberg (Red.) *Biophysics of consciousness: A foundational approach.* New York: World Scientific: 129–148.

Solms, M. (2017c) What is 'the unconscious', and where is it located in the brain? A neuropsychoanalytic perspective. *Annals of the New York Academy of Sciences*, 1406: 90–97.

Solms, M. (2018a) Review of A. Damasio, 'The Strange Order of Things'. *Journal of the American Psychoanalytic Association,* 66: 579–586.

Solms, M. (2018b) The scientific standing of psychoanalysis. *British Journal of Psychiatry – International,* 15: 5–8.

Solms, M. (2018c) The neurobiological underpinnings of psychoanalytic theory and therapy. *Frontiers in Behavioral Neuroscience*, 12(294): 1–12.

Solms, M. (2019a) The hard problem of consciousness and the Free Energy Principle. *Frontiers in Psychology,* 10: 2714. doi:10.3389/fpsyg.2018.02714.

Solms, M. (2019b) Does one size fit all? https://www.therapyroute.com/article/psychoanalysis-does-one-size-fit-all-by-m-solms

Solms, M. (2020) New project for a scientific psychology: General scheme. *Neuropsychoanalysis*, 22(1–2): 5–35.

Solms, M. (2021a) Dreams and the hard problem of consciousness. In: S. Della Salla (Red.) *Encyclopedia of behavioral neuroscience.* New York: Oxford University Press: 678–686.

olms, M. (2021b) Notes on some technical terms whose translation calls for comment. In: M. Solms (Red.) *Revised standard edition of the complete psychological works of Sigmund Freud*, 24. Lanham: Rowman & Littlefield (to be published)

Solms, M. (2021d) *De verborgen bron. Reis naar de oorsprong van het bewustzijn.* The hidden spring. Journey to the source of consciousness. Amsterdam: Bezige Bij.

Solms, M. (2021e) Revision of drive theory. *JAPA,* 69(6): 1033–1091.

Solms, M. (2021f) A Revision of Freud's Theory of the Biological Origin of the Oedipus Complex. *The Psychoanalytic Quarterly*, 90(4): 555–581.

Solms, M., & Saling, M. (1986) On psychoanalysis and neuroscience: Freud's attitude to the localizationist tradition. *International Journal of Psychoanalysis,* 67: 397-416.

Solms, M., & Saling, M. (1990) *A moment of transition: Two neuroscientific articles by Sigmund Freud.* Londen: Karnac.

Solms, M., & Turnbull, O. (2002) *The brain and the inner world: An introduction to the neuroscience of subjective experience.* London: Karnac.

Solms, M., & Turnbull, O. (2011) What is neuropsychoanalysis? *Neuropsychoanalysis*, 13: 133–145.

Solms, M., & Panksepp, J. (2012) The id knows more than the ego admits. *Brain Sciences*, 2: 147–175.

Solms, M., & Zellner, M. (2012) Freudian drive theory today. In: A. Fotopoulou, D. Pfaff & M. Conway (Red.) *From the couch to the lab: Trends in psychodynamic neuroscience.* New York: Oxford University Press: 49–63.

Solms, M., & Friston, K. (2018) How and why consciousness arises: Some considerations from physics and physiology. *Journal of Consciousness Studies*, 25: 202–238.

Spitz, R. A. (1945) Hospitalism—an inquiry into the Genesis of psychiatric conditions in early childhood. *Psychoanalytic Study of the Child*, 1: 53–74.

Stern, D. (1985) *The interpersonal world of the infant: A view from psychoanalysis and developmental psychology.* New York: Basic Books.

Stern, D. N. (1995) *The motherhood constellation: A unified view of parent-infant psychotherapy.* New York: Basic Books.

Stern, D. N., Sander, L. W., Nahum, J. P., Harrison, A. M., Lyons-Ruth, K., Morgan, A. C., & Tronick, E. Z. (1998) Non-interpretive mechanisms in psychoanalytic therapy: The something more than interpretation. *International Journal of Psycho-Analysis*, 79: 903–921.

Stortelder, F., & Ploegmakers-Burg, M. (2010) Adolescence and the reorganization of infant development: A neuro-psychoanalytic model. *Journal of the American Academy of Psychoanalysis* 38: 503–531.

Strauss, C.-L. (1962) *La Pensée Sauvage.* Paris: Plon.

Strozier, C. B. (2001) *Heinz Kohut: The making of an analyst.* London/New York: Other Press.

Swaab, D. (2010) *We zijn ons brein. Van baarmoeder tot Alzheimer.* Amsterdam: Atlas/Contact.

Symington, N. (1986) *The analytic experience.* London: Free Association Books.

Teuber, H.-L. (1955) Physiological psychology. *Annual Review of Psychology*, 6: 267–296.

Thorndike, E. (1911) *Animal intelligence: Experimental studies.* London: Macmillan.

Thys, M. (2006) Beter worden van waarheid [Getting better from truth]. *Tijdschrift voor Psychoanalyse*, 12(2): 136–142.

Thys, M. (2015a) Tussenhuids [In between skins]. *Tijdschrift voor Psychoanalyse*, 21(2): 146–148.

Thys, M. (2015b) Projectieve identificatie tussen doodsdrift en intersubjectiviteit [Projective identification between death drive and intersubjectivity]. *Tijdschrift voor Psychoanalyse*, 21: 83–97.

Thys, M. (2023) Tussen verwonding en verwondering. Over trauma, herhalingsdwang en doodsdrift. (Between Injury and Amazement. On trauma, repetition compulsion and death drive. In: Franckx, C. & Hebbrecht, M. (Red.) *Het kinderlijk trauma. Verloren tussen tederheid en passie.* (Childhood Trauma. Lost between Tenderness and Passion). Antwerpen/'s Hertogenbosch: Gompel & Svacina.

Tronson, N. C., & Taylor, J. R. (2007) Molecular mechanisms of memory reconsolidation. *Nature Reviews Neuroscience*, 8(4): 262–275.

Turnbull, O. H., Zois, E., Kaplan-Solms, K., & Solms, M. (2006). The developing transference in amnesia: Changes in interpersonal relationship, despite profound episodic-memory loss. *Neuropsychoanalysis*, 8(2): 199–204.

Tsakiris, M., & Critchley, H. (2016) Interoception beyond homeostasis: Affect, cognition and mental health. *Philosophical Transactions of the Royal Society B: Biological Sciences*, 371(1708): 20160002.

Twain, M. (1970) *Man is the only animal that blushes ... or needs to. The wisdom of Mark Twain.* New York: Stanyan Books, Random House.

Tzara, T. (1975) Manifeste sur l'amour faible et l'amour amer. In: H. Béhar (Ed.) Œuvres Complètes, tome I {1912–*1924)*: texte établi, présenté et annoté par. Paris: Flammarion.

Vaillant, G. E. (1995) *The wisdom of the ego.* Cambridge: Harvard University Press.

Vandenberghe, J. (2009) De neurowetenschappen, een zegen voor de psychotherapie? [The neurosciences, a blessing for psychotherapy?]. *Tijdschrift voor Psychotherapie*, 35(1): 18–24.

Vandenberghe, J., Van Oudenhove, L., & Cuypers, S. E. (2010) Wat doet psychotherapie met het brein? Een niet-reductionistische 'neurofilosofische' visie [What psychotherapy does with the brain? A non-reductionist neurophilosophical view]. *Tijdschrift voor Psychiatrie*, 2010(7): 455–462.

Vanheule, S. (2011) *The Subject of Psychosis: A Lacanian Perspective.* Hampshire: Palgrave Macmillan. https://doi.org/10.1057/9780230355873.

Vansina-Cobbaert, M. (1993) Per-agir. *Revue Belge de Psychanalyse*, 23: 13–31.

Verhaeghe, P. (1991) *Klinische psychodiagnostiek vanuit de discourstheorie* [Clinical psychodiagnostics inspired by discourse theory]. Gent: Idesça.

Verhaeghe, P. (1998) Trauma and Hysteria within Freud and Lacan. *THE LETTER* 14: 87–106.

Verhaeghe, P. (2001) Subject and body: Lacan's Struggle with the Real. In: P. Verhaeghe (Ed.) *Beyond gender: From subject to drive.* New York: Other Press: 65–97.

Verhaeghe, P. (2002) *Over normaliteit en andere afwijkingen.* Leuven/Leusden: Acco.

Verhaeghe, P. (2004) *On being normal and other disorders: A manual for clinical psychodiagnostics.* New York: Other Press.

Verhaeghe, P. (2009) *Het einde van de psychotherapie* [The end of psychotherapy]. Amsterdam: Bezige Bij.

Verhaeghe, P. (2010) Geestdrift voor het brein [Enthusiasm for the brain]. In: M. Kinet & A. Bazan (Red.) *Psychoanalyse en neurowetenschap: de geest in de machine* [Psychoanalysis and neuroscience: The ghost in the machine]. Antwerpen/Apeldoorn: Garant: 59–77.

Verhaeghe, P. (2012) *Identiteit* [Identity]. Amsterdam: De Bezige Bij.

Verhaeghe, P. (2015) *Autoriteit* [Authority]. Amsterdam: De Bezige Bij.

Verhaeghe, P. (2017) Trauma en hysterie bij Freud en Lacan [Trauma and hysteria in Freud and Lacan]. *Tijdschrift voor Psychoanalyse*, 2: 86–97.

Verhaeghe, P. (2022) *Intieme vreemden* [Intimate Strangers]. Amsterdam: Lemniscaat.

Verhaeghe, P., & Declercq, F. (2002) Lacan's goal of analysis: Le sinthome or the feminine way. In: L. Thurston (Ed.) *Re-Inventing the symptom: Essays on the final Lacan.* New York: Other Press: 59–83.

Verhaest, S., Pierloot, R., & Janssens. L. (1982) Comparative assessment of two different types of therapeutic communities. *International Journal of Social Psychiatry*, 28(1): 46–52. https://doi.org/10.1177/002076408202800106.

Vermote, R. (2015) Een geïntegreerd psychoanalytisch model in het licht van enkele neurowetenschappelijke bevindingen [An integrated psychoanalytical model in the light of some neuroscientific findings]. *Tijdschrift voor Psychoanalyse & haar toepassingen*, 21(1): 3–12.

Vermote, R. (2018) *Reading Bion.* New York/London: Routledge.

Vermote, R., & Vansina-Cobbaert, M. J. (2019) A psychoanalytic hospital unit for people with severe personality disorders. In S. Frisch, R. D. Hinshelwood, D. Houzel &

J. Pestalozzi (Eds.) *Psychoanalytic psychotherapy in institutional settings.* London/New York: Routledge: 75–93.

Verschuere, B., Crombez, G., & Koster, E. (2001) The international affective picture system. *Psychology Belgica*, 41: 205–217.

Vijver, Van de G., Bazan, A., & Detandt, S. (2017) The mark, the thing, and the object: On what commands repetition in Freud and Lacan. *Frontiers in Psychology*, 8: 2244. https://doi.org/10.3389/fpsyg.2017.02244.

Vleminck, De J. (2014) Een kleine genealogie van de doodsdrift: autopsie van een voetnoot in 'Aan gene zijde van het lustprincipe' [A small genealogy of the death drive: Autopsy of a footnote in Beyond the pleasure principle]. *Tijdschrift voor Psychoanalyse*, 20(1): 23–36.

Waal, De F. (2017) *Are we smart enough to know how smart animals are?* London: Faber & Faber.

Watt, D. F., & Panksepp, J. (2009) Depression: An evolutionarily conserved mechanism to terminate separation distress? A review of aminergic, peptidergic, and neural network perspectives. *Neuropsychoanalysis*, 11(1): 7–51.

Wei Zhang, Qi Pan, & Benyu Guo (2022) The significance of infant research for psychoanalysis. *Humanities and social sciences communications*, 9: 194.

Weisberg, D. S., Keil, F. C., Goodstein, J., Rawson, E., & Gray, J. R. (2008) The seductive allure of neuroscience explanations. *Journal of cognitive neuroscience*, 20(3): 470–477.

Westen, D., Gabbard, G. O., Westen, D., & Gabbard, G. O. (2002) Developments in cognitive neuroscience: I. Conflict, compromise, and connectionism. *Journal of the American Psychoanalytic Association*, 50(1): 53–98.

Winnicott, D. W. (1984 [1956]) Primary maternal preoccupation. In: D. W. Winnicott (Ed.) *Through paediatrics to psychoanalysis: Collected papers.* London: Karnac: 300–305.

Winnicott, D. W. (1990 [1960]) Theory of the parent-infant relationship. In: *The maturational process and the facilitating environment.* London: Karnac Books: 46.

Winnicott, D. W. (1971) Playing: A theoretical statement. In: *Playing and reality.* London: Tavistock.

Withers, R. (2008) Descartes' dreams. *Journal of Analytical Psychology*, 53(5): 691–709.

Wrangham, R., & Peterson, D. (1998) *Agressieve mannetjes — Over mensapen en de oorsprong van geweld bij de mens* [Aggressive males – On great apes and the origin of violence in man]. Amsterdam: Nieuwezijds.

Yalom, I. D. (1980) *Existential psychotherapy.* New York: Basic Books.

Yovell, Y., Solms, M., & Fotopoulou, A. (2015) The case for neuropsychoanalysis: Why a dialogue with neuroscience is necessary but not sufficient for psychoanalysis. *The International Journal of Psychoanalysis*, 96(6): 1515–1553.

Yu, C. K. (2001a) Neuroanatomical correlates of dreaming: The supramarginal gyrus controversy (dream work). *Neuropsychoanalysis*, 3: 47–60.

Yu, C. K. (2001b) Neuroanatomical correlates of dreaming. II: The ventromesial frontal region controversy (dream instigation). *Neuropsychoanalysis*, 3: 193–202.

Zeh, J. (2010 [2007]) *Speeldrift* [Play drive]. Amsterdam: Ambo/Anthos.

Zenoni, A. (1991) *Le corps de l'être parlant. De l'évolutionnisme à la psychanalyse.* Bruxelles: De Boeck.

Žižek, S. (1989) *The sublime object of ideology.* London: Verso.

Žižek, S. (1992 [1991]) *Looking awry: An introduction to Jacques Lacan through popular culture.* New York: MIT Press.

Žižek, S. (1997) *Het subject en zijn onbehagen* [The ticklish subject]. Amsterdam: Boom.

Žižek, S. (2006) *The parallax view.* Cambridge/London: MIT Press.

Index

Note: Page numbers followed by "n" denote endnotes.

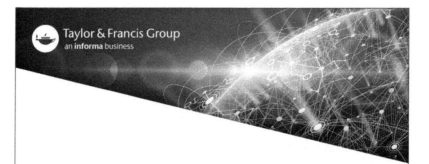